The Perspectives of People with Dementia

of related interest

Hearing the Voice of People with Dementia
Opportunities and Obstacles
Malcolm Goldsmith
Preface by Mary Marshall
ISBN 1 85302 406 6

Including the Person with Dementia in Designing and Delivering Care
'I Need to Be Me!'
Elizabeth Barnett
Foreword by Mary Marshall
ISBN 1 85302 740 5

The Spiritual Dimensions of Ageing
Elizabeth MacKinlay
ISBN 1 84310 008 8

Primary Care and Dementia
Steve Iliffe and Vari Drennan
Foreword by Murna Downs
ISBN 1 85302 997 1

Healing Arts Therapies and Person-Centered Dementia Care
Edited by Anthea Innes
ISBN 1 85302 038 X

Drug Treatments and Dementia
Stephen Hopker
ISBN 1 85302 760 X

User Involvement and Participation in Social Care
Research Informing Practice
Edited by Hazel Kemshall and Rosemary Littlechild
ISBN 1 85302 777 4

Younger People with Dementia
Planning, Practice and Development
Edited by Sylvia Cox and John Keady
Foreword by Mary Marshall
ISBN 1 85302 588 7

The Perspectives of People with Dementia

Research Methods and Motivations

Edited by Heather Wilkinson

Jessica Kingsley Publishers
London and Philadelphia

First published in the United Kingdom in 2002 by
Jessica Kingsley Publishers Ltd,
116 Pentonville Road, London
N1 9JB, England
and
325 Chestnut Street,
Philadelphia PA 19106, USA.

www.jkp.com

© Copyright 2002 Jessica Kingsley Publishers Ltd

Library of Congress Cataloging in Publication Data
A CIP catalog record for this book is available from the Library of Congress

British Library Cataloguing in Publication Data
A CIP catalogue record for this book is available from the British Library

ISBN 1 84310 001 0

Printed and Bound in Great Britain by
Athenaeum Press, Gateshead, Tyne and Wear

Contents

Part one: Ethical and practical issues of involvement

1   Including people with dementia in research: methods and motivations   9
Heather Wilkinson, University of Stirling

2   Getting down to brass tacks: a discussion of data collection
with people with dementia   25
Charlotte L. Clarke, University of Northumbria at Newcastle
and John Keady, University of Wales, Bangor

3   Ethical issues in dementia care research   47
Helen Bartlett and Wendy Martin, Oxford Dementia Centre,
Oxford Brookes University

4   Including the perspectives of older people in institutional care during the consent process   63
Gill Hubbard, University of Stirling, Murna Downs,
University of Bradford, and Susan Tester, University of Stirling

5   Including people with dementia: advisory networks and user panels   83
Lynne Corner, University of Newcastle

Part two: The views of people with dementia

6   Should people with Alzheimer's disease take part in research?   101
Elaine Robinson

7   Did research alter anything?   109
James McKillop

Part three: Methods and motivations

8   Working with staff to include people with dementia
    in research   117
    Kate Allan, University of Stirling

9   Successes and challenges in using focus groups with
    older
    people with dementia   139
    Claire Bamford, Centre for Health Services Research and Institute
    for Ageing and Health, University of Newcastle and Errollyn Bruce,
    Bradford Dementia Group, University of Bradford

10 'Nobody's ever asked how I felt'   165
    Rebekah Pratt, University of Stirling

11 Don't leave me hanging on the telephone: interviews
    with people with dementia using the telephone   183
    Anne Mason and Heather Wilkinson, University of Stirling

12 Using video observation to include the experiences
    of people with dementia in research   209
    Ailsa Cook, University of Stirling

13 South Asian people with dementia: research issues   223
    Alison M. Bowes and Heather Wilkinson, University of Stirling

    LIST OF CONTRIBUTORS   243

    SUBJECT INDEX   247

    AUTHOR INDEX   253

Ethical and Practical Issues of Involvement

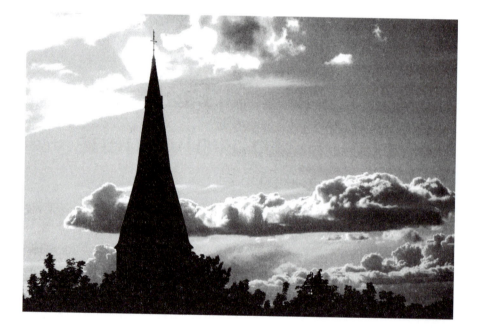

Including people with dementia in research
Methods and motivations

Heather Wilkinson

As probably one of the most excluded groups in society, people with dementia experience the double jeopardy (Rodeheaver and Datan 1988) of being older people with a cognitive impairment. For women this experience can be even more isolating and exclusionary (Proctor 2001) in a society where ageism and stigma against people with mental health issues reflect deep power inequalities in the relationships between individuals and wider society. Recent work with older people in general has attempted to address such imbalances, especially between service users and health care professionals (Beresford and Harding 1993). Despite this increased recognition of the need for older people to retain and maintain choice and control in their lives (Nusberg 1995), people with dementia remain a silent and excluded voice. With recent moves in policy and practice emphasising social inclusion and justice (Adults with Incapacity (Scotland) Act 2000; Scottish Executive 1999), perhaps it is timely to examine the position of people with dementia in social research. To what extent have we developed effective motivations and methods through which the experiences and views of people with dementia can be included in and inform research, policy and practice contexts?

This chapter focuses on three key questions: *should* we be including people with dementia in social research on dementia; *can* we include them; and what still needs to be done to facilitate work in this area?

Should we be including people with dementia in research?

During the development of several research projects that included people with dementia as participants[1] I was often asked 'why bother?' or 'is it possible?' These questions usually came from other researchers, members of ethics committees and health and social care practitioners. In response to these questions and from discussion with other people in the field of dementia research and care, several reasons emerged. The first, broadest reason for why we should include people with dementia themselves is the basic requirement to shift the power inequalities inherent in some research on and with people with dementia (Reed and Payton 1998). Amongst several other reasons, closely linked to this first one, was that we need to develop an understanding of the experience of living with dementia and this understanding cannot really be developed from proxy reports.

Shifting power

In order to begin to address the power inequalities in the relationships between people with dementia and others, it is essential to reduce and remove the stigma associated with the disease. Assuming people with dementia cannot participate in research or are unable to share views and experiences is a reinforcement of negative stereotypes of incapacity. Historically, images and perceptions of people with dementia are based on the traditional stereotype of senile old people who have 'lost their mind' (Lyman 1998; Mills 1997; Sabat 1998; Sabat and Harre 1994). This stereotypical and negative approach to people with dementia reinforces their marginalisation.

The place of dementia as a disease category has had an important impact on the way society sees people with dementia. Despite the first published case of dementia appearing in the early 1900s (by Alois Alzheimer 1907) it was not until the mid-1970s, when shifts in demographics and an ageing population became of concern, that the largely economic significance of dementia created more interest. This rise in interest was reflected in a corresponding increase in funding for dementia research. The search for cause and cure had begun and understanding of research tended to be grounded in a medical model portraying those with dementia as diseased brains rather than individual people (Cheston and Bender 1999). Such a social construction of a disease (Harding and Palfrey 1997, p.4) with medical professionals as the architects, results in a perpetuation of stigma, excess disability (Brody 1971) and unequal relations that relegate people with dementia to 'lesser' or 'other'.

Any approach aimed at reducing these negative effects requires a fundamental change in the way that people with dementia are thought about, so they can be seen as people who have valid experiences and whose behaviours are driven by meaning (Sabat 1994). In the wider field of disability research, this approach is offered through the social model of disability (Barnes 1992; Oliver 1992), a concept currently starting to inform dementia care and research (Downs and Wilkinson 1999; Proctor 2001). A social model approach argues that social relations between people and within society are fundamental to the experiences of disabled people. Rather than focusing on individual medical problems or deficits, this approach highlights the impact of social and environmental barriers, cultural processes and policy frameworks that actively and systematically disable people. From a research perspective, the social model of disability has also added to our thinking and challenged assumptions around how research is conducted and in particular highlights research conducted in more inclusive ways that challenge the traditional 'social relations of research production' (Oliver 1992).

Attitudinal, policy and environmental factors certainly increase the disability experienced by people with dementia. One way to challenge and reduce these factors is to develop a better understanding of what it means to be a person with dementia living in a society with these barriers and how the power relations can be changed. However, conducting research that might provide some of this information requires a direct engagement with people with dementia themselves. This means directly addressing various issues about research principles and design. Again the issue of power relations is central. It is necessary to make these relations clearly visible and to engage in a reflexivity that questions the basis of such relations (Harding 1991; Wilkinson and Kitzinger 1996). Power in research extends beyond researcher/researched and into their relative positions in society, for example older people experience ageism through frequently applied negative stereotypes (Bytheway 1995; Jack 1995). Dementia research can learn from both feminist and disability research, where the problems of how to do research 'with' rather than 'on' people have already been grappled with (Duelli Klein 1983; Riddell, Wilkinson and Baron 1998; Rioux and Bach 1994).

In engaging with these issues, research that attempts to be more democratic and inclusive has tended to be described as participatory or emancipatory. The main underpinnings to emancipatory and participatory research have been described as:

> Conventional relationships, whereby the researcher is the 'expert' and the researched merely the object of investigation are inequitable...people have the right to be consulted about and involved in research which is involved in issues affecting their lives. (Stalker 1988, p.6)

However, there are important differences between the two types of approach:

> In emancipatory research the research processes themselves and the outcomes of the research are part of the liberation of disabled people – that is part of the process of changing society to ensure their full-time participation and citizenship. This is not just a process of empowerment as in participatory research, where research participants may be given opportunities to tell their own stories and analyse their own situation, but in terms of disabled people taking control of the research processes which shape their lives. (French and Swain 1997, p.28)

In reality the difficulties in engaging in more emancipatory research often result in a slide into more participatory research (Walmsley 2001) and I return to this point later in the chapter.

Developing understanding

One way to challenge current inequalities in social relations for people with dementia is to develop more inclusive research strategies in order to gather the experiences and views of people with dementia themselves, rather than (or in addition to) those of proxies.

Challenging the medicalised view by a more person-centred focus on the individual experience of living with a memory impairment (Cotrell and Schulz 1993; Downs 1997) is perhaps best exemplified in the first steps towards building services and policy that are based on and responsive to personal needs and experiences. How can service providers and policy makers know what people with dementia want and need without being able to gather and include their views and experiences? Lyman has outlined a model that acknowledges the importance of social factors such as individual variation, autonomy, negotiation, and the effects of power relationships in dementing illnesses. Her work indicates that people with dementia are social actors who live with impairment and interact with others in caregiving relationships within a variety of socially structured environments (Lyman 1989, p.604).

That these subjective experiences can be accessed is increasingly acknowledged: 'There is a distinction between the cognitive self which may be affected by memory loss and the experiencing feeling self which may be much less impaired' (Froggatt 1988, p.133).
Underpinning the need to engage with people with dementia are debates around the individual's self of sense; their rights; and the value to be gained from a concern with their perspectives (Downs 1997). On the whole research in this area has been driven by the imperative to 'include the voices' of service users in evaluations of services and there have been very recent and promising attempts to include the perspectives of people with dementia (Barnett 2000).

These debates are a reflection of, and are reflected in, recent government policy. The role of older people in the planning and delivery of care has been emphasised in recent years (Thompson and Thompson 2001; Thornton and Tozer 1994). The introduction of community care throughout the 1980s/90s (Department of Health 1990) focused on empowering individuals, in a service user sense, to become effective 'consumers' within a wider context of active citizenship (Barnes 1997). A result of the rhetoric around individuals as consumers has been the creation of a tension between 'empowering' individuals to make choices and excluding people who do not have the ability or support to make their voices heard within the unequal power relations inherent in accessing services. In reality, individuals experiencing these policies are probably not the 'ideal' citizen/ consumer/decision maker upon which the policies are predicated. Recent claims discussing the success of social care markets in England highlight the need for 'better information holdings' to improve the effectiveness of social care markets and service delivery based on 'services that users need and want' (Knapp *et al.* 2001, p.305).

There are also moral and practical risks in not engaging in a more person-centred, inclusive approach (see for example Sabat 1998). The greatest risk is what wider society and services miss in *not* having the subjective experiences of individuals living with the illness:

> We are at risk of not delivering adequate care to our patients and their families. If we do not get to know our patients' experience of the illness beyond the results of medical, cognitive and functional tests and assessments, our clinical decisions will not represent patient needs equitably. (Cohen 1991, p.7)

Currently for people with dementia our ways of 'knowing' what people with dementia need and want remain limited and exclusionary.

In summary, several positive reasons emerge from the debate around the question of whether we should include the perspectives and experiences of people with dementia themselves. On a wider level it is important to shift the power inequalities in relations with people with dementia, and start to reduce and challenge the stigmatised and stereotypical views held. In order to do so it is essential to have a greater understanding of personal experience as opposed to the medically and socially constructed images and perceptions that currently prevail:

> The reliance upon the biomedical model to explain the experience of dementing illness overlooks the social construction of dementia and the impact of treatment contexts and care giving relationships on disease progression. (Lyman 1989, p.597)

In addition, to ensure that the voices of people with dementia do inform policy and practice it is essential to find ways of hearing and privileging their voices, as emphasised in the policy moves that focus on user involvement. To increase our factual information on what helps and hinders quality of life and inclusion for people with dementia, and to have an understanding of what it means to live with dementia, we have to be able to access the personal experiences of individuals who are actually living with dementia. In the next part of this chapter I examine our current methodological issues and ask Can we include people with dementia?

Can we include people with dementia?

Despite promising calls for a more inclusive approach (Cotrell and Schulz 1993; Downs 1997) and several strong reasons for including people with dementia, this has been slow to happen. Inclusion/exclusion can be seen as both concepts and processes. A person can be described as excluded when he/she is 'geographically resident in a society and he/she does not participate in the normal activities of citizens in that society' (Burchardt, Le Grand and Piachaud 1999, p.230).

Participating in activities that are valued by others; having some decision-making powers; and being able to draw support from family, friends and others in a wider community can be seen as important indicators of social inclusion (Burchardt, Le Grand and Piachaud 1999, p.230). People with dementia have identified all of these as areas or activities they become excluded from following a diagnosis of dementia (Keady 1996; Mason and Wilkinson 2001; Pratt and Wilkinson 2001; Proctor 2001). Taking part in research that could inform service development, policy or practice could also be seen as an important normal activity, yet people with dementia are again rarely involved in work of this type.

A central reason for the lack of research that includes people with dementia is the limited and fragmented understanding and experience of methods that are known to enable the voice of the person to be safely and effectively encouraged, heard and understood. Until very recently the perception that people with dementia were unable to express feelings, opinions and views was widely held. This exclusionary view that assumed people with dementia could not be included is slowly being challenged as the practical difficulties of *how* to include people with dementia are gradually overcome.

Stalker, Gilliard and Downs (1999) note that many methods and concerns can be transferred from the field of learning disabilities to dementia research, especially in relation to the use of qualitative methods and processes for consent. In most cases of recent social research on dementia, methods chosen have been qualitative in order to explore subjective experience of individuals (Gillies 1995; Keady 1999; Pratt and Wilkinson 2001). Two key issues have emerged from attempts to engage in more inclusive research: the impact of individual cognitive ability on participation; and the negotiated social relations necessary for the safe participation of people with dementia.

Cognitive abilities

One of the main concerns around gathering the perspectives of people with dementia has been the impact of their degree of cognitive impairment. Influential work in the past has been carried out by Lyman (1998) that challenges the idea that only mildly impaired people can participate (see also Moniz-Cook *et al.* 1998). Work exploring the narrative identity of people with dementia (Mills 1997) also found that people with moderate to severe cognitive impairment could recall emotional memories. Wells and Dawson (2000) in a study of 112 male veterans with dementia in the USA found that individuals retained abilities in the areas of self care, social, interactional and interpretative abilities, although abilities relating to self care and activities of daily living were retained longer than those of recall and language. Furthermore, the abilities of individuals varied considerably, consistent with evidence pertaining to cognitive changes in dementia (Wells and Dawson 2000), meaning that participation is very much an individual concern. In addition to taking part in recent research projects, people with dementia have attempted to describe directly their lived experiences (Davis 1998; McGowin 1993). All this work highlights that people with dementia *do* have the ability to participate in research. There are certain issues relating specifically to cognitive decline that are particular to people with dementia, but progressive decrease in cognitive ability associated with dementia should not be seen as a criterion for exclusion from research studies. In fact it provides a strong motivation for searching for innovative and exploratory ways in which their views can be heard.

Social relations and participation

A result of the push to gather the views of service users is the rise in the number of service evaluations that attempt to include people with dementia (Cheston, Bender and Byatt 2000). Work done has included the use of questionnaires and structured interviews; semi-structured interviews; observation; and focus groups (Barnett 2000; Brooker 1995; Davis 1998; Smallwood 1997; Sperlinger and McAuslane 1994). The issue of power inherent in the social relations experienced by people with dementia is implicit in all of these methods. Research aimed at privileging the voices of the older people has to engage with these power inequalities inherent in the research principles and design. The relative positions of marginalised people in society (such as older people and the ageism they experience) can be reflected in the researcher/researched dynamic. Whilst it is essential to include the views of people with dementia it is also important to recognise and take account of these inherent power inequalities and allow care and time to enable people to participate fully (or not as they choose).

Moving forwards

This book is a first attempt to bring together first-hand reports on projects that have tried to include the perspectives of people with dementia and it explores methods that may facilitate more inclusionary practices. The book is intended to provide an informative and accessible exploration of the controversial and changing factors significant in the inclusion of people with dementia in social research. Many of the contributors have brought knowledge and experience from other areas, in particular the fields of learning disability and gerontology. Each chapter in this book reports on the experience gleaned from actual projects that sought to include and focus on the views and experiences of people with dementia.

The collection begins with a useful and comprehensive review, by Charlotte Clarke and John Keady, of recent studies that have attempted, through a variety of methods, to ascertain the view of people with dementia. The first part of the book goes on to focus in more depth on some of the practical and ethical issues relating to including people with dementia. Helen Bartlett and Wendy Martin discuss a range of key ethical issues that arise when undertaking research with people with dementia. Gill Hubbard, Murna Downs and Sue Tester engage in an exploration of consent issues, focusing on assessing the ability of potential participants to give informed consent, and discuss strategies for involving people with dementia unable to give informed consent.

I mentioned earlier the problem encountered when attempting more participatory research and how this often results in a slide into more participatory research (Walmsley 2001). The chapter by Lynne Corner is a useful example and discussion of an attempt to make research more emancipatory and to involve people with dementia in the agenda setting and as advisors to research.

The second part of the book is perhaps the most important – two people with dementia who have participated in research studies have contributed chapters. Both Elaine and James are living with dementia and have been involved in research reported in one of the chapters in the book. Their chapters report on their personal views and experiences of research and address the issues of whether people with dementia should and can be included in research. Not only do these chapters illustrate yet another way in which people with dementia can be included, they present powerful and articulate examples of the necessity and importance of ensuring such inclusion.

The chapters in the third part of the book each detail a different method used to ascertain the views of individuals with dementia. From early work with people with dementia in focus groups (Bamford with Bruce) and face-to-face interviews (Pratt) to the challenges of telephone interviews with people with dementia (Mason and Wilkinson) and the progress in using video to gather data (Cook), the difficulties and rewards of working with people with dementia are highlighted.

Many of the chapters highlight the importance and benefits of developing research relationships with people with dementia. Rebekah Pratt focuses on the role of 'gatekeepers' and how they can provide support and assistance when including people with dementia. Claire Bamford (with Errollyn Bruce) also explores the research relationship in their chapter describing focus groups with people with dementia. The challenges of building a research relationship are also highlighted in the chapter by Anne Mason and Heather Wilkinson, which explores the practicalities and possibilities of telephone interviews with people with dementia. Ailsa Cook, in her chapter on videos, aimed to gather the experiences of people with moderate and advanced dementia, whose views have largely been excluded due to lack of knowledge about how to interact with people with often profound communication difficulties. People from minority ethnic groups also tend to experience additional exclusion and the chapter by Alison Bowes and Heather Wilkinson explores some of the reasons that this has been the case for South Asian people with dementia.

The work reported here is innovative and exploratory but a lot of work remains to be done. Rather than an end I would like to see this book as a beginning – for more work that aims to include and involve people with dementia, and that increases awareness of how this can be done in a way that is safe to both researcher and researched but also in a way that privileges the voices, views and experiences of people with dementia. Many of the chapters in this book grapple with why and how to include people with dementia in positive ways, but the field of dementia research has a long way to go!

What still needs to be done?

It is clear that we have only come so far on a journey of discovery. The moral question of 'should we?' is in part answered by culminating experience and the outcomes of reflection and dissemination of pieces of work and also in part by people with dementia themselves who have taken part in research projects and dissemination (see for example the chapters by Robinson and McKillop in this book). However, it is also important to keep sight of the ethical issues surrounding inclusive and participatory research. No one should simply go out and talk to people with dementia – there are complex and sensitive issues to be overcome first. Overall, dementia research has a lot to learn from the experiences and motivations behind disability research, especially methods and motivations that are more participatory and emancipatory.

As yet there is no cure or effective treatment for everyone with dementia, so we have an imperative to focus on quality of life and the experiences, views and opinions of those people living with the disease. In this way we can move on from early and essential work focusing on evaluation and using proxy voices, to other ways of exploring and challenging, at a deeper and wider level, the attitudes and processes which can reduce stigma and bring people with dementia more inclusively into society. It is only by increasing our understanding of the lives they are living and their own personal experiences of living with dementia that the barriers to participation can be reduced.

In research there is always something else to be done and certainly in the area of methodology we have a long journey ahead. The projects reported here have involved important and often ground-breaking work, yet having achieved this level successfully there are still important directions, methods and issues to be explored. In particular there are the explorations still to be had around how to include people with more severe cognitive impairments who may be experiencing the later stages of the illness. We also need to be more aware of how dementia research can be made more participatory. Not only is progression to inclusionary research an essential requirement for the development of services that meet the needs of individuals, it is an ethical and moral underpinning on which dementia research can move forwards (Post 1998; Sabat 1998). I hope this book, by capturing a collection of current and very active social research which is inclusive of people with dementia, will help promote this belief and facilitate a shift in practice.

Acknowledgements

My favourite train journey is between Newcastle and Edinburgh. Both starting point and destination (whichever direction I happen to be travelling) have such positive associations for me and great scenery along the way.

It is also a journey with close associations with this book. The idea for this book occurred during one of those train rides. On previous trips I had often spent the travel time trying to think of ways around some of the difficulties I was having including people with dementia in some of my projects. The last three years working in the field of dementia research likewise have been a positive journey with some great scenery along the way: meeting and working with people with dementia; hearing about and sharing the ideas involved in the other projects reported in this book; and looking forwards to reaching the destination of producing a book that will help bring together what we have learned so far and highlight future routes and destinations.

I would like to express my sincere thanks to everyone who contributed to this book, often at short notice and with great enthusiasm and good will. In particular I would like to thank James McKillop and Elaine Robinson for sharing such personal and inspiring chapters. The support and patience of Amy Lankester-Owen, Claudia Conway and Jessica Kingsley during my trek into the unfamiliar territory of book editing deserves special thanks. To Ann, Andy, family and friends in both Edinburgh and Newcastle, thanks for being there and giving me reason to travel.

Note

1   The author is based at the Centre for Social Research on Dementia and has been grant-holder on several projects that were developed to include the person with dementia in research.

References:

Adults with Incapacity (Scotland) Act (2000) Scottish Executive, http://www.scottish. parliament.uk/parl.pdf.

Alzheimer, A. (1907) 'Uber eine eigernatige Erkrankung der Hirnrinde.' *Allgeneine Z. Psychiatrie 64*, 146.

Barnes, C. (1992) 'Qualitative research: Valuable or irrelevant?' *Disability, Handicap and Society 7*, 2, 115–124.

Barnes, M. (1997) *Care, Communities and Citizens.* London: Routledge.

Barnett, E. (2000) *Including People with Dementia in Designing and Delivering Care.* London: Jessica Kingsley Publishers.

Beresford, P. and Harding, T. (1993) (eds) *A Challenge to Change: Practical Experiences of Building User-Led Services.* London: NISW.

Brody, E. (1971) 'Excess disabilities of mentally impaired aged: Impact of individualized treatment.' *Gerontologist 25*, 1, 124–133.

Brooker, D. (1995) 'Looking at them looking at me. A review of observational studies into the quality of institutional care for elderly people with dementia.' *Journal of Mental Health 4*, 145–156.

Burchardt, T., Le Grand, J. and Piachaud, D. (1999) 'Social Exclusion in Britian 1991–1995.' *Social Policy and Administration 33*, 3, 227–244.

Bytheway, B. (1995) *Ageism.* Buckingham: Open University Press.

Cheston, R. and Bender, M. (1999) *Understanding Dementia: The man with the worried eyes.* London: Jessica Kingsley Publishers.

Cheston, R., Bender, M. and Byatt, S. (2000) 'Involving people who have dementia in the evaluation of services: A review.' *Journal of Mental Health* 9, 5, 471–479.

Cohen, D. (1991) 'The subjective experience of Alzheimer disease – the anatomy of an illness as perceived by patients and their families.' *The American Journal of Alzheimer's Care and Related Disorders and Research* May/June, 6–11.

Cotrell, V. and Schulz, R. (1993) 'The perspective of the patient with Alzheimer's disease: A neglected dimension of dementia research.' *Gerontologist 33*, 205–211.

Davis, R. (1998) *My Journey into Alzheimer's Disease.* Amersham: Scripture Press.

Department of Health (1990) *Care in the Community: Making it happen.* London: HMSO.

Downs, M. (1997) 'The emergence of the person in dementia research.' *Ageing and Society* 17, 597–607.

Downs, M. and Wilkinson, H. (1999) 'Dementia as a Disability: Towards a research agenda.' Paper presented at the Gerontological Society of America Annual Conference, San Francisco, 20–23 November.

Duelli Klein, R. (1983) 'How to do what we want to do: the ethics and politics of interviewing women.' In C. Bell and H. Roberts *Social Researching: Politics, Problems and Practice.* London: Routledge and Kegan Paul.

French, S. and Swain, J. (1997) 'Changing disability research: Participatory and emancipatory research with disabled people.' *Physiotherapy 83*, 1, 26–32.

Froggatt, A. (1988) *Self-Awareness in Early Dementia.* Open University Press Paper 16.

Gillies, B. (1995) 'The Subjective Experience of Dementia. A qualitative analysis of interviews with Dementia sufferers and their carers, and the implications for service provision.' Unpublished report. Tayside Health Board.

Harding, S. (1991) *Whose Science? Whose Knowledge? Thinking from Women's Lives.* Milton Keynes: Open University Press.

Harding, N. and Palfrey, C. (1997) *The Social Construction of Dementia: Confused Professionals?* London: Jessica Kingsley Publishers.

Jack, R. (1995) (ed.) *Empowerment in Community Care.* London: Chapman and Hall.

Keady, J. (1996) 'The experience of dementia: A review of the literature and implications for nursing practice.' *Journal of Clinical Nursing 5*, 275–288.

Keady, J. (1999) *The Dynamics of Dementia: A modified grounded approach theory study.* Unpublished PhD thesis. Bangor: University of Wales.

Knapp, M., Hardy, B., and Farder, J. (2001) 'Commissioning for Quality: Ten years of social care markets in England.' *Journal of Social Policy 30*, 2, 283–306.

Lyman, K. A. (1989) 'Bringing the social back in: A critique of the biomedicalisation of dementia.' *Gerontologist 29*, 597–605.

Lyman, K. A. (1998) 'Living with AD: The creation of meaning among persons with dementia.' *Journal of Clinical Ethics 9*, 1, 49–57.

Mason, A. and Wilkinson, H. (2001) 'The characteristics of people with dementia who are users and non-users of the legal system: A feasibility study.' Final Report to the Scottish Executive. Stirling.

McGowin, D. F. (1993) *Living in the Labyrinth: A personal journey through the maze of Alzheimer's.* Cambridge: Mainsail Press.

Mills, M. (1997) 'Narrative identity and dementia: A study of emotion and narrative in older people with dementia.' *Ageing and Society 17*, 673–698.

Moniz-Cook, E., Agar, S., Gibson, G., Win, T. and Wang, M. (1998) 'A preliminary study of the effects of early intervention with people with Dementia and their families in a memory clinic.' *Ageing and Mental Health 2*, 3, 199–211.

Moody, H. R. (1985) 'Issues of equity in the selection of subjects for experimental research in senile dementia of AT.' In V. L. Melnick and N. N. Dubler (eds) *AD: Dilemmas in clinical research.* Clifton NJ: Humana Press.

Murray, A., Furnish, S. and Lewis, N. (1996) 'Listening to people with dementia.' *Signpost* December, 13–14.

Nusberg, C. (1995) 'Preface.' In D. Thurz, C. Nusburg and J. Prather (eds) *Empowering Older People : An International Perspective.* London: Cassell.

Oliver, M. (1992) 'Changing the social relations of research production?' *Disability, Handicap and Society 7*, 2, 101–14.

Post, S. G. (1998) 'The fear of forgetfulness: A grassroots approach to an ethics of AD.' *Journal of Clinical Ethics 9*, 1, 71–80.

Pratt, R. and Wilkinson, H. (2001) 'The effect of being told the diagnosis of dementia from the perspectives of the person with dementia.' Final Report to the Mental Health Foundation. Stirling: CSRD.

Proctor, G. (2001) 'Listening to older women with dementia.' *Disability and Society. 16*, 3, 361–376.

Reed, J. and Payton, V. R. (1998) 'Privileging the voices of older service users: A methodological challenge.' *Social Sciences in Health 4*, 4, 230–242.

Riddell, S., Wilkinson, H. and Baron, S. (1998) 'From emancipatory research to focus group: People with learning difficulties and the research process. In P. Clough and L. Barton (eds) *Articulating with Difficulty: Research Voices in Inclusive Education.*, pp.78–95. London: Paul Chapman Publishing Ltd.

Rioux, M. And Bach, M. (1994) *Disability is not Measles: New research paradigms in disability.* Ontario: L'Institute Rocher.

Rodeheaver, D. and Datan, N. (1988) 'The challenge of double jeopardy – toward a mental health agenda for aging.' *American Psychologist 43*, 8, 648–654.

Sabat, S. R. (1994) 'Excess disability and malignant social psychology: A case study of AD.' *Journal of Community and Applied Psychology 4*, 3, 157–66.

Sabat, S. R. (1998) 'Voices of AD Sufferers: A call for treatment based on personhood.' *Journal of Clinical Ethics 9*, 1, 35–48.

Sabat, S.R. and Harre, R. (1994) 'The construction and deconstruction of self in AD.' *Ageing and Society 12*, 4, 443–461.

Scottish Executive (1999) *Making the Right Moves: Rights and Protection for Adults with Incapacity.* Edinburgh: Scottish Executive.

Scottish Office (1999) *Social Inclusion: Opening the Door to a Better Scotland.* Edinburgh: HMSO.

Smallwood, J. (1997) *Initial Report on Obtaining the Views of Activities Undertaken while in Care from People with Dementia.* Mental Health Services for Older Adults, Quality Department, Birmingham.

Sperlinger, D. and McAuslane, L. (1994) 'Listening to the views of users of services for people with dementia.' *Clinical Psychology Forum 73*, November, 2–4.

Stalker, K. (1998) 'Some ethical and methodological issues in research with people with learning difficulties.' *Disability and Society 13*,1, 5–13.

Stalker, K., Gilliard, J. and Downs, M. (1999) 'Eliciting user perspectives on what works.' *International Journal of Geriatric Psychiatry 14*, 120–134.

Thompson, N. and Thompson, S. (2001) 'Empowering older people: Beyond the care model.' *Journal of Social Work 1*, 1, 61–76.

Thornton, P. and Tozer, R. (1994) *Involving Older People in the Planning and Reviewing of Community Care: A Review of Initiatives.* York: Social Policy Research Unit.

Walmsley, J. (2001) 'Normalisation, emancipatory research and inclusive research in learning disability.' *Disability and Society 16*, 2, 187–295.

Wells, D. L. and Dawson, P. (2000) 'Description of retained abilities in older persons with dementia.' *Research in Nursing and Health 23*, 158–168.

Wilkinson, S. and Kitzinger, C. (1996) (eds) *Representing the Other.* London: Sage.

Chapter Two

Getting down to brass tacks
A discussion of data collection with people with dementia

Charlotte L. Clarke and John Keady

Introduction

This chapter aims to explore some of the main concepts surrounding data collection, ethical practice and social research conducted with people with dementia and their support networks, an agenda that has gathered real momentum from the mid-1980s and captured many new insights into the experience of those with dementia. In order to explore the philosophical and practical shift behind this movement, the chapter will commence by briefly rehearsing recent trends that have seen the person with dementia become the focal point of policy, research and practice attention. The chapter will then couple exemplars from the social science literature with the authors' own research experience to illuminate the varying facets of social research enquiry that have involved people with dementia, focusing in particular upon the data collection phase of the study. This aspect of the text will also be supported by literature from other fields that have experienced the marginalisation of people from research (such as people with learning disabilities and children). There are many points of overlap between the fields, notably in the approach to sensitive interviewing and ensuring informed consent to participate. Finally, the authors will conclude the chapter by pulling together the common threads from the provided accounts and outline a résumé of good practice in data collection that concerns people with dementia.

Dementia as a lived experience

Quite some time ago now, Gilleard (1984) in his seminal text on community care for people with dementia, noted the 'as yet unattended problems of the mildly or questionably dementing elderly population' (p.41). This position was also acknowledged in an earlier report by the Royal College of Physicians (1981), with the text suggesting that improved diagnostic practice in mild dementia would open up the possibility of preventative action and 'effective therapeutic intervention' (p.153). Whilst this is a laudable aim, it was uncertain at the time how it could be achieved as the health service provision for dementia care was invested in 'bricks and mortar', with buildings for continuing care, respite and day hospital provision dominating the landscape of service provision. Couple this lack of investment in primary care with a burgeoning social science literature that focused on the stress and burden of family carers (for comprehensive reviews see: Knight, Lutzky and Macofsky-Urban 1993; Kuhlman *et al.* 1991), and it is easy to see how people with dementia became distanced from their own experience and packaged as a future 'problem' for care agencies (Health Advisory Service 1982). Moreover, the 1980s saw few attempts to involve the person with dementia in the design, planning, implementation or evaluation of their own service provision, or to act as a research guide to help interpret the lived experience of the person with dementia.

However, from this rather negative appraisal, the shoots of a more inclusive research, practice and policy agenda were beginning to emerge. For instance, a report prepared for the King's Fund Centre (1986) in the UK brought together some key academics and policy makers who had a vested interest in the well-being of the person with dementia. At its heart their report set out an empowering agenda that attempted to view people with dementia, first and foremost, as individuals, and as people with legitimate access to services, as these five 'key principles' illustrate (King's Fund Centre 1986, p.7–8 abridged):

1. People with dementia have the same human value as anyone else irrespective of their degree of disability or dependence;

2. People with dementia have the same varied human needs as anyone else;

3. People with dementia have the same rights as other citizens;

4. Every person with dementia is an individual; and

5. People with dementia have the right to forms of support which do not exploit family and friends.

By spelling out such person-centred values the report was saying, in effect, that it was not people with dementia who were the 'problem' facing planners, providers and policy makers, but ageist attitudes and the inflexible nature of service design (King's Fund Centre 1986). On the other hand, the report did not actually contain any examples where such principles were applied to practice, and this omission may well have diminished its overall impact. Indeed, in the context of community care in the UK for people with dementia, it would be some time before such a positive service delivery could be reported in the literature with any degree of confidence (see Challis *et al.* 1997).

In part the catalyst for this service re-orientation and focus on the person with dementia emerged from the introduction of the NHS and Community Care Act (Department of Health 1990) and its emphasis upon user consultation and the negotiation of a mutually agreed package of care. Commenting at the time upon the impact of the community care reforms for people with dementia and their 'care manager', Winner (1993) suggested that this reform opened up a new challenge for the social work profession. Specifically, the legislation forced social workers, in their care manager role, to commence a dialogue with the person with dementia and record his/her needs and wants over and above those with whom he/she was living. Winner (1993) also argued that on-going assessment, enduring relationships and commitment were necessary if the person's sense of involvement with care agencies was to develop in any meaningful way, a finding reminiscent of that of Gilleard (1984). Moreover, Winner (1993) noted that the skills needed by social work staff to achieve this dialogue with people with dementia were at a very early stage of their development, and that progress was unlikely to be made without attention to the educational preparation of practitioners.

If the foundations for a heightened sensitivity and more inclusive practice agenda for people with dementia were laid in the NHS and Community Care Act (Department of Health 1990), they were cemented in subsequent policy initiatives, such as:

> mental illness targets set out in the White Paper *The Health of a Nation: A Strategy for Health in England* (Department of Health 1992) which included a focus on vascular dementia
>
> right for information on a diagnosis as part of the Patient's Charter (Welsh Office 1991)
>
> improvement of multi-agency working through the setting of 'action checklists' to challenge current practice with people with dementia and their families, for instance through the establishment of joint training initiatives and the sharing of the diagnosis of dementia with the person him/herself (Social Services Inspectorate/Department of Health 1996)
>
> better community response to older people living alone with mental health problems, particularly those with dementia (Alzheimer's Disease Society 1994; Social Services Inspectorate/Department of Health 1997)
>
> necessity of improving standards of care across the spectrum of service provision, including user consultation and carer support (Audit Commission 2000; Department of Health 1999; Health Advisory Service 2000, 1999).

In England, the UK Government has recently published the *National Service Framework for Older People* which, for the first time, sets national standards of care for both health and social services (Department of Health 2001). The National Service Framework (NSF) is underpinned by four main themes: respecting the individual; intermediate care; providing evidence-based specialist care; and promoting an active and healthy life.

Eight national standards then underpin these themes, and standard 7 focuses on the mental health needs of older people, with people with dementia and their carers being afforded considerable attention in the development of the strategy. Whilst a critique of the NSF is beyond the scope of this chapter, the strategy promotes the general benefits of an early diagnosis of dementia and the subsequent sharing of the diagnosis with the person with dementia.

Whilst this attention could be considered a cause for celebration, this optimism must be tempered, as a recent Audit Commission (2000) report identified a number of competing concerns in relation to the early identification and diagnosis of dementia. For instance, the report revealed that in a survey of general practitioners across the 12 study sites in the sample (n = 1000+), only 52 per cent of respondents believed it important to make an early diagnosis of dementia; a point quantified in the report with the following example: 'What is the point in looking for an untreatable illness?' (Audit Commission 2000, p.21). Arguably, of even more concern than such nihilistic attitudes, was the finding that only 44 per cent of general practitioners in the sample used any specific tests or protocols to help them diagnose dementia. Whilst words are vital weapons in the development of a more inclusive, sensitive and person-centred culture, for people with dementia it is crucial that the rhetoric is turned into meaningful change on both a practice footing (De Lepeleire and Heyrman 1999) and in the investment of training for general practitioners (Milne *et al.* 2000).

All in all there remains much to be done to encourage primary care teams to look sensitively at the needs of people with dementia, and for service planners to begin to fund a comprehensive dementia care service within each regional health authority. As the Audit Commission (2000) report identified, where memory clinics exist within a locality, rates of early referral and detection improved. With the National Institute of Clinical Excellence recently accepting the efficacy of anti-Alzheimer medication, the arguments continue to be strengthened for the availability of a range of early diagnostic and specialist support services to augment the work of the general practitioner and primary care team (Downs *et al.* 2000; Fortinsky, Leighton and Wasson 1995). This support extends to the availability of 'memory change' guidelines to enhance the efficacy of cognitive screening (Trickey *et al.* 1998).

In practice this move towards a more sensitive and inclusive approach to people with dementia was helped by the creative work of the Bradford Dementia Group in the UK and its driving emphasis upon person-centred values (Kitwood 1988, 1993, 1997; Kitwood and Bredin 1992a, 1992b). The persuasive arguments put forward by Kitwood and his colleagues, to see the person first and the dementia second, did much to raise awareness and stimulate an agenda for change, particularly on the need to challenge the 'malignant social psychology' that had surrounded the experience of dementia (Kitwood 1993, 1997). Crucially, this paradigm shift saw the person with dementia moved to the forefront of attention with service providers challenged to address inadequate care practices. In the work of the Bradford Dementia Group this re-orientation of service values was expressed through the development of the observational method of Dementia Care Mapping (DCM) (Kitwood and Bredin 1992a), although DCM is designed predominantly for use in residential care facilities as practice evaluations by Williams and Rees (1997), Brooker *et al.* (1998) and Younger and Martin (2000) attest. Accordingly, other approaches are required for intervention with people with early dementia, and initiatives that have built upon therapeutic work in this area include:

> facilitation of support groups (Cheston 1996; Duff and Peach 1994; Jackson and Wonson 1987; McAfee, Ruh and Bell 1989; Yale 1991)

> use of memory therapy in clinical practice (for a review see Clare 1999)

> use of psycho-social interventions in memory clinics (Moniz-Cook *et al.* 1998)

> benefits of using a dedicated counselling service around the time of diagnosis (Pinner 2000; Whitsed-Lipinska 1998), and the availability of specialist counselling services for younger people with dementia (Harvey *et al.* 1998)

application of life review approaches (Woods *et al.* 1992)

one-to-one engagement in psychotherapy (Orbach 1996), particularly the efficacy of cognitive behavioral therapy (see for example: Sutton 1994; Teri and Gallagher-Thompson 1991).

Arguably, despite this encouraging trend, these advances have still not permeated routine practice where a focus on the more traditional approaches to working with people with dementia, for instance through reality orientation, resolution or validation therapy (see respectively: Feil 1992a, 1992b; Holden and Woods 1988; Stokes and Goudie 1990) remains dominant (see also Normann, Asplund and Norberg 1999). On the other hand, the increasing emphasis placed upon understanding and responding to early dementia may well bring about the necessary re-orientation of intervention, skills and preparation for practice, as a recent study about advancing cognitive screening by nurse practitioners in primary care has demonstrated (Adams and Page 2000). Furthermore, the closer relationship between practice and people with early dementia places an additional layer of responsibility upon social researchers to conduct studies in such naturalistic settings, and it is to an appreciation of this role that the chapter will now turn.

Research and the person with early dementia: A focus on data collection

Early Steps

If such approaches are to continue to develop there is a need for greater understanding of dementia as it is personally experienced. This agenda has been taken forward most forcibly by people with early dementia themselves as their own stories and life experiences permeate our thinking and sensitivity to this area, as a recent text by Snyder (1999) so movingly illustrates. Prior to this movement, however, social scientists began to question the validity of studies that omitted the perspective of the person with dementia and started to search for its meaning through proxy accounts from carers. For instance, La Rue, Watson and Plotkin (1993) found that forgetfulness reported by carers was by far the most common early indicator of dementia, followed by: confusion; depression; agitation; inattention;

getting lost language; and motor problems. Whilst such data are potentially useful, they remain a second-hand account. Cotrell and Schulz (1993) were severely critical of this carer-focused agenda which, in their opinion, subjugated the person with Alzheimer's disease to '…an entity to be studied rather than someone who can directly contribute to an understanding of the illness and its course' (p.205).

Studies that have sought personal perspectives on early dementia have, to date, been confined to relatively small samples (see for example: Acton *et al.* 1999; Gillies 2000; Goldsmith 1996; Keady and Gilliard 1999; Nygård and Borell 1998; Phinney 1998; Wuest, Ericson and Stern 1994), a methodological standpoint that, perhaps, reflects the depth of understanding necessary to gain such perspectives. In one of the earliest reported social research studies on self-awareness in early dementia, Froggatt (1988) suggested that the social construction of memory failure be seen as an episodic mixture of forgetfulness over recent events, absent-mindedness and internal preoccupation with thoughts and daydreams. In this pioneering study Froggatt outlined 'formidable obstacles' (p.134) towards undertaking qualitative research with people with early dementia, embracing ethical, methodological and psychological considerations. Drawing on her own research methodology Froggatt (1988, p.134 slightly abridged) listed nine areas to consider in conducting qualitative research with people with early dementia, namely:

1.   The underlying morality of asking those who are already mentally precarious about aspects of themselves which it may be painful to contemplate.

2.   Gaining access to 'sufferers' [original text] can only be through a general practitioner, psychogeriatrician, community psychiatric nurse or social worker.

3.   Research probably needs to be conducted using a variety of methods: semi-structured conversations with the 'sufferer' [original text], additional interviews with key relatives and principal carer, and consulting records (with consent), to build up a psycho-biography.

4. Researchers/interviewers need to be experienced and/or trained, as interviews are likely to be emotionally difficult.

5. Funding may be difficult to obtain, in the light of prevailing ageism.

6. Gaining consent from the 'sufferer' [original text] to talk about his/her current life. If a person withholds consent because of anxiety this must be respected. Building trust, warmth and empathy during the encounter can reduce the anxiety for those who do consent.

7. There is reticence about conducting research in this area for fear of increasing anxiety. To legitimate the anxiety could be a way of strengthening the person's hold on reality.

8. Interviews with 'sufferers' [original text] may need to be relatively short and, if conducted more than once, spaced close together to benefit memory.

9. Interviews with relatives may need to be lengthy as they struggle to understand the minutiae of observed behaviour, trying instinctively to make sense of it.

Froggatt (1988) also acknowledged that it may be a positive step in the interview to ask the person with early dementia to go on taking risks, facing up to new experiences and 'to cope with the anxiety' (p.135). Moreover, she suggested that the researcher should engage in lateral thinking and feeling; implicitly, this acknowledges that the interview will have an emotional impact upon the interviewer and that this should be recognised in any prospective study design.

A second early insight into data collection with people with dementia was provided through a selection of the papers resulting from the Hughes Hall Project for Later Life (see: Pollitt 1994; Pollitt and Anderson 1991; Pollitt, Anderson and O'Connor 1991; and Pollitt, O'Connor and Anderson 1989), particularly Pollitt and Anderson's (1991) commendable honesty in admitting that during the study 'they did not always ask the right questions, or ask them to the right person' (p.30). Synthesising the 'methods' section of each of the papers stemming from the Hughes Hall Project for Later Life, we were able to identify a number of issues emerging from their overall study design and approach to data collection. Prime amongst these were that: interviews with people with early dementia could be undertaken both jointly with the carer and individually; relatives largely controlled their dependants' entry into the study, and placed their own meaning upon the value of the research process; satisfactions in caregiving were present at this early point in the caregiving trajectory; and at the beginning of an interview, it was crucial to build rapport and ask the right questions.

In their influential paper Cotrell and Schulz (1993) also highlighted a number of strategies in developing a study design for people with early dementia and these included the belief that:

> small sample sizes were appropriate
>
> people with dementia may feel less threatened if the study is undertaken in their own home
>
> the timing of the interview should be set by the person with early dementia, to enhance their feelings of control over the research process
>
> the perspective of the caregiver is a valuable source of information
>
> people with early dementia may welcome the opportunity to discuss their experiences.

The importance of this last statement should not be under-estimated as it serves as a reminder over ownership of 'dementia', and the need to be able to explore its meaning from a personal perspective and interpretation. However, in order to do justice to the experience of people with early dementia, one of the major issues facing social researchers is that of ensuring data quality and it is to this area that attention is now turned.

Data quality

We can understand some of the practical issues surrounding data collection with people with dementia by learning from other fields of work with marginalised groups. For example, Marquis and Jackson (2000) describe a study with 26 adults with disabilities (both physical and mental). Where they were concerned about the acquiescence of people with learning disabilities, in dementia care the concern might be with confabulation – in both cases there is concern about the stability of perspective of the individual and the accuracy of the information.

Marquis and Jackson (2000) tackled this concern through prolonged engagement with the individual (a minimum of two interviews) and questioning that allowed the repetition and confirmation of issues. Similarly, Knox, Mok and Parmenter (2000) in another study used repeated interviewing with people with learning disabilities.

At the heart of the data collection described by Knox *et al.* (2000) is a collaborative approach in which both the interviewer and the interviewee set the agenda for the interview, this being negotiated during the preceding interview. In this way, the authors of both studies describe having confidence in learning of the issues that concern those being interviewed, and argue that it is possible to elicit data that is confirmable and trustworthy from people with limited communication and cognitive abilities.

Fundamental to the collaborative approach adopted by Knox *et al.* (2000) is consideration of the credibility of the participants in the interview situation. For example, the interviewee must be framed as an expert if his/her views are to do more than serve to validate the interviewer's perceptions – there must be a genuine and determined effort to respect the interviewee as the master of his/her thoughts. Indeed, Keady and Gilliard (1999) report that during their interviews with people with dementia, people were often 'amazed that someone was taking an interest in their situation' (p.240). Knox *et al.* (2000) provide a further illustration of this phenomenon, this time from the learning disability field:

> Informants were more familiar with the role of passivity…in research as research subjects and in society as service recipients. Indeed, the focus on learning from these people, rather than about them took them from the realm of 'clienthood' to that of research partner or colleague. They were seen as experts in their own right. Their silenced voices were unsilenced. (p.58)

Similarly, Booth and Booth (1996) urge that 'researchers should put more emphasis on overcoming the barriers that impede the involvement of inarticulate subjects in narrative research instead of dwelling on their limitations as informants' (p.55). However, in our eagerness to accommodate the perspectives of people with dementia, the role of carers must not be neglected. Keady (1999) invited the participation of relatives as part of the interview process, although the introductory letter emphasised that the person living with early memory loss was to be the main focus of the interview. This approach was based upon the experience of Pollitt and Anderson (1991) and the presumption that:

> carers act as a gatekeeper to the person with early dementia

> protective caregiving would be evident at this time (see Bowers 1987)

> The early adjustment to dementia could be seen as a system of personal and family adaptation, with both perspectives being important to consider.

The interviewer must also have credibility in the eyes of the interviewee if the interviewee is to entrust the interviewer with access to the private domains of his/her life and thoughts (Lee 1993). Indeed, Knox *et al.* (2000) describe the credibility of their interviewer as deriving from their personal experiences of living with someone with a learning disability rather than from their research expertise.

Booth and Booth (1996) describe four styles of communication presented by people with learning disabilities, that challenge the pursuit of research. All of these points are transferable to working with people with dementia. First, inarticulateness in which language use is influenced by lack of self-esteem, social isolation and anxiety as well as language skills. Second, unresponsiveness in which open questions result in limited responses. Third, a concrete frame of reference, with difficulty generalising from experience and thinking in abstract terms (the very things required of someone being interviewed, as a rule). Fourth, problems with time such that it may be difficult for the interviewees to 'tell their story'. Booth and Booth suggest that an appropriate interviewing style is direct in its questioning, validating of the individual, reduces anxiety, and avoids asking about frequencies or time sequences.

The credibility of data collected can be strengthened in a number of ways. Deatrick and Faux (1991) and Sartain, Clarke and Heyman (2000) consider the ways of achieving this with young children as interviewees, another group whose voice has been neglected in the annals of research history. They emphasised the importance of using neutral territory during data collection, avoiding tiredness and anxiety, responding appropriately to emotional reactions during the interview, data recording reliability and augmentation of interviews.

The use of neutral territory, or by preference territory that is most familiar to the person with dementia, is important for both the point of collecting data and the point of recruitment into a study. It places the interviewee in a position of advantage, at least over the environment in which he/she is asked to make a decision about participation and engage in data collection. This would suggest that a memory clinic, for example, should be the least preferred location for recruitment and data collection and the individual's own home the location of preference. However, the process of identifying a group of people to approach about research involvement is usually achieved through their service contact. As a result, locations of service provision are where the initial approach and possibly data collection do indeed take place very often. For example, Robinson et al. (1997) interviewed eight younger people who were being assessed for dementia, with the interviews taking place in a room off the main ward in which they were staying for a few days for diagnostic assessment. Similarly, Keady (1999) recruited a sample of ten people with early dementia at the six-month follow-up appointment to a memory clinic.

The duration and pacing of an interview should be dictated by the interviewee to avoid tiredness and anxiety. For people with dementia, it is reasonable to assume that an interview would be of shorter duration than for someone who is not cognitively disabled. Keady (1999) restricted interviews to 45 minutes, although Robinson et al. (1997) reports interviewing younger people with dementia for an average of two hours. The event of an interview should be viewed as far more than the period that the tape-recorder is switched on. The lead-in period is essential to establishing the tone of the interview, allowing the individual to relax and a crucial time in which the interviewer communicates that the life of the interviewee is valued. It is during this period that cups of coffee may be offered and made, general exchanges about the weather or families made, and discussion about the purposes of the study and destination of the data reinforced (assuming here that there has been a preceding point of negotiation to recruit the individual to a study). Similarly, the period after the tape-recorder has been switched off is one of continuing interest in the person as an individual. Unnecessary haste in concluding and departing may result in the interviewee feeling 'used' and understandably reluctant to engage with subsequent periods of data collection. The period of actual data collection occupies, then, only part of the time available before tiredness enforces a conclusion to the exchange.

It is essential that the researcher validates the experiences and expressions of the person with dementia by responding appropriately to emotional reactions during the interview. This does of course bring some conflict to the research situation where it becomes impossible and inappropriate to maintain a conventional stance of detachment from the individual. Again, if the interview situation is understood as a shared encounter between the researcher and the interviewee, the emphasis moves away from detached data collection to a period of mutual learning and exchange. However, there may be times when the exchange transcends that which has been consented to, and when there is a need to be quite specifically 'therapeutic' in interaction (Raudonis 1992). Indeed, Keady (in Clarke and Keady 1996) describes turning off the tape-recorder during an interview to support the individual and then returning to the taped interview a little later. Such times are disallowed as research data if they are considered by both parties to have gone beyond public information into that which the individual wished to remain private (Field and Morse 1985). In this way, informed consent in research has to be understood as a process that is continually negotiated and that supplements the more conventional formal consenting process. Process consent is one of continual renegotiations and is particularly appropriate in social research where there is reflexivity between data to be collected and data already collected, and where participants may wish to place limits on the information that is available as research data (Knox *et al.* 2000; Raudonis 1992).

Data recording reliability is necessary to ensure an accurate and complete record of the research event. There are, of course, many technical aspects to the collection of any data including the effectiveness of a tape-recorder to pick up sound but not to be overwhelmed by extraneous noises (for example, passing traffic, background shouting). There is also a need to decide what 'counts' as data, and the standard interview privileges the spoken word in a way that may be inappropriate when doing research with people with dementia. For example, non-verbal communication may be crucial to an understanding of the meaning of the words spoken, or sounds may be very quiet or not distinguishable as formed words or sentences. In such situations, the observational skills of the researcher are emphasised to either augment a transcript of a tape-recorded interview or as data in its own right. The structured observational process of Dementia Care Mapping is well established, but it is more a model of collecting data about people rather than with them. An alternative observational approach was adopted by Cantley *et al.* (2000a, 2000b) to evaluate a small group home for younger people with dementia. All three tenants of the home had very poor verbal skills and the researcher spent many hours sitting in various locations in the home keeping extensive notes of people's activity and interactions. It was essential that this observational data collection was minimally intrusive (a challenge in the confines of a domestic home) and respected the dignity and privacy of the tenants. This was attempted by restricting data collection to one researcher over a short (six-week) period and by considerable pre-observation preparation of the people involved.

The standard research interview asks for information from interviewees that is both reflective and prospective (the referential function of interviews described by Booth and Booth 1996). This dependence on memory and anticipation renders this form of data collection unsuitable for people with dementia at times. However, measures can be taken to augment the interview with prompts or with devices to help people consider the topic of the interview. For example, Sartain *et al.* (2000), in a study of children with repeated hospital admissions, started each interview by asking the child to draw a picture of what it was like being at home and in hospital.

This drawing then became the focus of the interview. In an evaluation of a multidisciplinary team for younger people with dementia, Reed *et al.* (2000) were concerned that people with dementia would be unable to identify the team members with the services they received. During the interviews a photograph chart was used showing a head and shoulders photograph of each of the team members and the interviewer. The chart was simply lain on a suitable surface, for example a coffee table, in front of the interviewee and interviewer for the duration of the interview. This chart also detailed the key areas to be discussed during the interview, providing an easy-access memory board for people with dementia. This aided the discussion and was used by all the people with dementia and carers who were interviewed.

Conclusion

This chapter has focused on the details of managing data collection in social research with people with dementia. However, this activity has to be located in the context of the whole study design and the philosophical persuasions of the research team. There are a number of key issues about involving people with dementia in research but these are actually concerns that should influence the research encounter with anyone. Perhaps it is a reflection of our stage of engagement with people with dementia that we see them as a 'special case' for data collection at all. Accordingly, we would view the following criteria as crucial in helping to structure data collection with people with dementia:

> Data collection requires creativity and a positive approach to managing the challenges of researching with people with dementia.

> There must be opportunity for people to articulate and express their perspective in a way that, as researchers, we can have confidence in the data. This requires:

>> sufficient engagement to allow confirmation of issues raised, for example through repeated interviews

>> a mutually trusting relationship

a collaborative approach with the person with dementia, allowing a mutual process of agenda setting

minimising anxiety and tiredness, for example by considering the duration, pacing and location of data collection

augmentation of data collection, either through multiple corroborating sources or by structuring the data collection episode to maximise engagement.

The person must be valued, and know that they are valued, for their knowledge; this suggests that the researcher will need to be emotionally engaged with the individual.

Detailed attention must be paid to reliable data recording.

For people with dementia to be present only through the proxy voice of their carer, or by having research done unto them (with or even without their consent), is no longer a tenable position (Downs and Crossan 1999; McColgan, Valentine and Downs 2000). The challenge is with us as researchers to find effective and meaningful ways of engaging with people with dementia in the research situation. This is not just an abstract challenge – an inability to achieve this is to continue to deny ourselves access to the knowledge of people with dementia that might be usefully deployed in developing care. The cost of failing in this methodological agenda is not one that the future of dementia care can afford if we aspire to place the experience of the person at the forefront of thinking and practice.

References

Acton, G. J., Mayhew, P. A., Hopkins, B. A. and Yauk, S. (1999) 'Communicating with Individuals with dementia: The impaired person's perspective.' *Journal of Gerontological Nursing 25*, 2, 6–13.

Adams, T. and Page, S. (2000) 'New pharmacological treatments for Alzheimer's disease: Implications for dementia care nursing.' *Journal of Advanced Nursing 31*, 5, 1183–1188.

Alzheimer's Disease Society (1994) *Home Alone: Living alone with dementia* London: Alzheimer's Disease Society.

Audit Commission (2000) *Forget Me Not: Mental health services for older people.* London: Audit Commission.

Booth, T. and Booth, W. (1996) 'Sounds of silence: Narrative research with inarticulate subjects.' *Disability and Society 11*, 1, 55–69.

Bowers, B. J. (1987) 'Inter-generational caregiving: Adult caregivers and their ageing parents.' *Advances in Nursing Science 9*, 2, 20–31.

Brooker, D., Foster, N., Banner, A., Payne, M. and Jackson, L. (1998) 'The efficacy of Dementia Care Mapping as an audit tool: Report of a 3-year British NHS evaluation.' *Aging and Mental Health 2*, 1, 60–70.

Cantley, C., Smith, M., Clarke, C. and Stanley, D. (2000a) *An Independent Supported Living House for People with Early Onset Dementia: Evaluation of a Dementia Care Initiative Project.* Newcastle upon Tyne: Dementia North.

Cantley, C., Reed, J., Stanley, D., Clarke, C., Banwell, L. and Capel, S. (2000b) 'Early onset team proves a success.' *Journal of Dementia Care 8*, 4, 10–11.

Challis, D., von Abendorff, Brown, P. and Chesterman, J. (1997) 'Care Management and Dementia: An evaluation of the Lewisham Intensive Case Management Scheme.' In S. Hunter (ed) *Dementia: Challenges and New Directions*, pp.139–164. London: Jessica Kingsley.

Cheston, R. (1996) 'Stories and metaphors: Talking about the past in a psychotherapy group for people with dementia.' *Ageing and Society 16*, 5, 579–602.

Clare, L. (1999) 'Memory rehabilitation in early dementia.' *Journal of Dementia Care 7*, 6, 33–38.

Clarke C. L. and Keady J. (1996) 'Researching dementia care and family caregiving - extending ethical responsibilities.' *Health Care in Later Life 1*, 2, 85–95.

Cotrell, V. and Schulz, R. (1993) 'The perspective of the patient with Alzheimer's disease: A neglected dimension of dementia research.' *Gerontologist 33*, 2, 205–211.

De Lepeleire, J. and Heyrman, J. (1999) 'Diagnosis and management of dementia in primary care at an early stage: The need for a new concept and an adapted procedure.' *Theoretical Medicine and Bioethics* 20, 215–228.

Department of Health (1990) *NHS and Community Care Act.* London: HMSO.

Department of Health (1992) *The Health of a Nation: A Strategy for Health in England.* London: HMSO.

Department of Health (1999) *Caring About Carers: A National Strategy for Carers.* London: The Stationery Office.

Department of Health (2001) *National Service Framework for Older People.* London: The Stationery Office.

Deatrick, J. A. and Faux, S. A. (1991) 'Conducting qualitative studies with children and adolescents.' In J. M. Morse (ed) *Qualitative Nursing Research: A Contemporary Dialogue*, pp.185–203. Newbury Park, CA: Sage.

Downs, M. and Crossan, B. (1999) 'Trading places: New challenges for research in nursing and residential homes.' *Aging and Mental Health 3*, 1, 8–9.

Downs, M., Cook, A., Rae, C. and Collins, K. E. (2000) 'Caring for patients with dementia: The GP perspective.' *Aging and Mental Health 4*, 4, 301–304.

Duff, G. and Peach, E. (1994) *Mutual Support Groups: A Response to the Early and Often Forgotten Stage of Dementia.* Report. Stirling, Dementia Services Development Centre: University of Stirling.

Feil, N. (1992a) *V/F Validation The Feil Method: How To Help Disorientated Old-Old.* Second Edition. Cleveland, Ohio: Edward Feil Productions.

Feil, N. (1992b) 'Validation therapy with late-onset dementia populations.' In G. Jones and B. M. L. Miesen (eds) *Caregiving In Dementia: Research And Applications*, pp.199–218. London: Routledge.

Field P. A. and Morse J. M. (1985) *Nursing Research: The Application of Qualitative Approaches*. London: Chapman and Hall.

Fortinsky, R. H., Leighton, A. and Wasson, J. H. (1995) 'Primary care physicians' diagnostic, management, and referral practices for older persons and families affected by dementia.' *Research on Aging 17*, 2, 124–148.

Froggatt, A. (1988) 'Self-awareness in early dementia.' In B. Gearing, M. Johnson and T. Heller (eds) *Mental Health Problems in Old Age: A Reader*, pp.131–136. Buckingham: Open University Press.

Gilleard, C. J. (1984) *Living With Dementia: Community Care of the Elderly Mentally Infirm*. London: Croom Helm.

Gillies, B.A. (2000) 'A memory like clockwork: Accounts of living through dementia.' *Aging and Mental Health 4*, 4, 366–374.

Goldsmith, M. (1996) *Hearing the Voice of People with Dementia: Opportunities and Obstacles*. London: Jessica Kingsley Publishers.

Harvey, R., Rossor, M. N., Skelton-Robinson, M. and Garralda, E. (1998) *Young Onset Dementia: Epidemiology, clinical symptoms, family burden, support and outcome*. London: NHS Executive.

Health Advisory Service (1982) *The Rising Tide*. Surrey: NHS, Sutton.

Health Advisory Service 2000 (1999) *Standards for Mental Health Services for Older People*. Health Advisory Service and Pavilion Publishing: Brighton.

Holden, U. P. and Woods, R. T. (1988) *Reality Orientation: Psychological Approaches to the 'Confused' Elderly*. Second Edition. Edinburgh: Churchill Livingstone.

Jackson, D. and Wonson, S. (1987) 'Alzheimer's re-socialization: A group approach towards improved social awareness among Alzheimer's patients.' *American Journal of Alzheimer's Care and Related Disorders and Research 2*, 5, 31–35.

Keady, J. (1999) *The Dynamics of Dementia: A Modified Grounded Theory Study*. Unpublished PhD thesis. University of Wales, Bangor.

Keady, J. and Gilliard, J. (1999) 'The early experience of Alzheimer's disease: Implications for partnership and practice.' In T. Adams and C. Clarke (eds) *Dementia Care: Developing Partnerships in Practice*, pp.227–256. London: Baillière Tindall.

King's Fund Centre (1986) 'Living well into old age: Applying principles of good practice to services for people with dementia.' Report Number 63. London: King's Fund Publishing Office.

Kitwood, T. (1988) 'The technical, the personal and the framing of dementia.' *Social Behaviour 3*, 161–180.

Kitwood, T. (1993) 'Person and Process in Dementia.' *International Journal of Geriatric Psychiatry 8*, 541–545.

Kitwood, T. (1997) *Dementia reconsidered: The Person Comes First*. Buckingham: Open University Press.

Kitwood, T. and Bredin, K. (1992a) 'A new approach to the evaluation of dementia care.' *Journal of Advances in Health and Nursing Care 1*, 5, 41–60.

Kitwood, T. and Bredin, K. (1992b) 'Towards a theory of dementia care: Personhood and well-being.' *Ageing and Society. 12*, 269–287.

Knight, B. G., Lutzky, S. M. and Macofsky-Urban, F. (1993) 'A Meta-analytic review of interventions for caregiver distress: Recommendations for future research.' *Gerontologist 33*, 2, 240–248.

Knox, K., Mok, M. and Parmenter, T. R. (2000) 'Working with the experts: Collaborative research with people with an intellectual disability.' *Disability and Society 15*, 1, 49–61.

Kuhlman, G. J., Wilson, H. S., Hutchinson, S. A. and Wallhagen, M. (1991) 'Alzheimer's disease and family caregiving: Critical synthesis of the literature and research agenda.' *Nursing Research 40*, 6, 331–337.

La Rue, A., Watson, J. and Plotkin, D. A. (1993) 'First symptoms of dementia: A study of relatives reports.' *International Journal of Geriatric Psychiatry 8*, 239–245.

Lee, R. M. (1993) *Doing Research on Sensitive Topics.* London: Sage.

Marquis, R. and Jackson, R. (2000) 'Quality of life and quality of service relationships: Experiences of people with disabilities.' *Disability and Society 15*, 3, 411–425.

McAfee, M. E., Ruh, P. A. and Bell, P. (1989) 'Including persons with early stage Alzheimer's disease in support groups and strategy planning.' *American Journal of Alzheimer's Care and Related Disorders and Research 4*, 6, 18–22.

McColgan, G., Valentine, J. and Downs, M. (2000) 'Concluding narratives of a career with dementia: Accounts of Iris Murdoch at her death.' *Ageing and Society 20*, 97–109.

Milne, A. J., Woolford, H. H., Mason, J. and Hatzidimitriadou, E. (2000) 'Early diagnosis of dementia by GPs: An exploratory study of attitudes.' *Aging and Mental Health 4*, 4, 292–300.

Moniz-Cook, E., Agar, S., Gibson, G., Win, T. and Wang, M. (1998) 'A preliminary study of the effects of early intervention with people with dementia and their families in a memory clinic.' *Aging and Mental Health 2*, 3, 199–211.

Normann, H. K., Asplund, K. and Norberg, A. (1999) 'Attitudes of registered nurses towards patients with severe dementia.' *Journal of Clinical Nursing 8*, 353–359.

Nygård, L. and Borell, L. (1998) 'A life-world of altering meaning: Expressions of the illness experience of dementia in everyday life over 3 years.' *Occupational Therapy Journal of Research 18*, 2, 109–136.

Orbach, A. (1996) *Not Too Late: Psychotherapy and Ageing.* London: Jessica Kingsley Publishers.

Phinney, A. (1998) 'Living with dementia from the patient's perspective.' *Journal of Gerontological Nursing 24*, 6, 8–15.

Pinner, G. (2000) 'Truth-telling and the diagnosis of dementia.' *British Journal of Psychiatry 176*, 514–515.

Pollitt, P.A. (1994) 'The meaning of dementia to those involved as carers.' In F. A. Huppert, C. Brayne and D. W. O'Connor (eds) *Dementia and Normal Aging,* pp.257–271. Cambridge: Cambridge University Press.

Pollitt, P. A. and Anderson, I. (1991) 'Research methods in the study of carers of dementing elderly people: Some problems encountered in the Hughes Hall Project for later life.' *Generations: Bulletin of the British Society of Gerontology 16* (Summer), 29–32.

Pollitt, P. A., Anderson, I. and O'Connor, D. W. (1991) 'For better or for worse: The experience of caring for an elderly dementing spouse.' *Ageing and Society 11*, 443–469.

Pollitt, P. A., O'Connor, D. W. and Anderson, I. (1989) 'Mild Dementia: Perceptions and problems.' *Ageing and Society 9*, 261–275.

Raudonis, B. M. (1992) 'Ethical considerations in qualitative research with hospice patients.' *Qualitative Health Research 2*, 2, 238–249.

Reed, J., Cantley, C., Stanley, D., Clarke, C., Banwell, L. and Capel, S. (2000) *An Evaluation of the Lewis Project: A Service for people with Early Onset Dementia*. Newcastle upon Tyne: Centre for Care of Older People.

Robinson, P., Ekman, S., Meleis, A. I., Winblad, B. and Wahlund, L. (1997) 'Suffering in silence: The experience of early memory loss.' *Health Care in Later Life 2*, 2, 107–120.

Royal College of Physicians (1981) 'Organic mental impairment in the elderly: Implications for research, education and the provision of services. A report of the Royal College of Physicians by the College Committee on Geriatrics.' *Journal of the Royal College of Physicians of London 15*, 3, 141–167.

Sartain, S., Clarke, C. L. and Heyman, R. (2000) 'Hearing the voices of children with chronic illness.' *Journal of Advanced Nursing 32*, 4, 913–921.

Snyder, L. (1999) *Speaking Our Minds: Personal reflections from Individuals with Alzheimer's*. New York: W.H. Freeman and Co.

Social Services Inspectorate/Department of Health (1996) *Assessing Older People With Dementia in the Community: Practice Issues for Social and Health Services*. Wetherby: HMSO.

Social Services Inspectorate/Department of Health (1997) *Older People With Mental Health Problems Living Alone: Anybody's Priority?* Wetherby: HMSO.

Stokes, G. and Goudie, F. (eds) (1990) *Working with Dementia*. Bicester, Oxon: Winslow Press.

Sutton, L. J. (1994) 'What It Is To Lose One's Mind.' Paper presented at the 10th International Conference of Alzheimer's Disease International, Edinburgh.

Teri, L. and Gallagher-Thompson, D. (1991) 'Cognitive behavioural interventions for treatment of depression in Alzheimer's patients.' *Gerontologist 31*, 3, 413–416.

Trickey, H., Harvey, I., Wilcock, G. and Sharp, T. (1998) 'Formal consensus and consultation: A qualitative method for development of a guideline for dementia.' *Quality in Health Care 7*, 192–199.

Welsh Office (1991) *Health: A Charter for Patients in Wales*. Cardiff, Welsh Office: HMSO.

Whitsed-Lipinska, D. (1998) 'Counselling services for people with dementia.' *Journal of Dementia Care 6*, 5, 10–11.

Williams, J. and Rees, J. (1997) 'The use of "dementia care mapping" as a method of evaluating care received by patients with dementia – an initiative to improve quality of life.' *Journal of Advanced Nursing 25*, 316–323.

Winner, M. (1993) 'User choice, care management and people with dementia.' Paper presented at the British Society of Gerontology Annual Research Conference, Norwich.

Woods, B., Portnoy, S., Head, D. and Jones, G. (1992) 'Reminiscence and life review with persons with dementia: Which way forward?' In G. Jones and B. M. L. Miesen (eds) *Caregiving in Dementia: Research and Applications*, pp.137–161. London: Routledge.

Wuest, J., Ericson, P. K. and Stern, P. N. (1994) 'Becoming strangers: The changing family caregiving relationship in Alzheimer's disease.' *Journal of Advanced Nursing 20*, 437, 443.

Yale, R. (1991) *A Guide to Facilitating Support Groups for Newly Diagnosed Alzheimer's Patients.* San Francisco: Alzheimer's Association.

Younger, D. and Martin, G. W. (2000) 'Dementia care mapping: An approach to quality audit for services for people with dementia in two health districts.' *Journal of Advanced Nursing 32*, 5, 1206–1212.

Chapter Three

Ethical issues in dementia care research

Helen Bartlett and Wendy Martin

Introduction

Research into the health and social aspects of dementia is increasing as the number of people with dementia in the UK continues to rise. As the predominant medical discourses that previously surrounded a person with dementia have been challenged (Bond and Corner 2001), the focus of research now increasingly aims to promote an understanding of how people with dementia construct their social worlds, and participants are viewed as active participants in the research process (Clarke 1999; Crossan and McColgan 1999). Goldsmith (1996) argues about the importance of hearing the 'voice' of the person with dementia and research now increasingly aims to understand their subjective experiences. Whilst this important change is welcomed it has, at the same time, raised new ethical and methodological dilemmas for researchers in dementia care. These issues have been addressed in relation to clinical research (see Agarwal *et al.* 1996; Baskin *et al.* 1998; Berghmans 1998; Berghmans and Ter Meulen 1995; High 1993;) and researchers are now starting to explore the ethical dilemmas associated with social research (Adams and Clarke 1999; Clarke and Keady 1996; Crossan and McColgan 1999; Downs 1997; Kayser-Jones and Koenig 1994; Stalker, Duckett and Downs 1999; Stalker, Gilliard and Downs 1999).

This chapter sets out to explore the key ethical issues in dementia research, drawing on lessons from a study about empowering older people with dementia.[1] It will set out the approaches adopted in relation to these complex issues and some of the debates and challenges surrounding them. Further, the ethical implications of involving older people with dementia as active participants in the research process will be explored.

Ethical principles

The key ethical principles to be followed in any research involving human participants are well documented (see for example Kayser-Jones and Koenig 1994). First, it is necessary to ensure that research participants have consented to their involvement. The elements of consent have been identified as: the information given, the capacity to understand it and the voluntariness of any decision taken (Medical Research Council 1991). The process of informed consent not only involves establishing rights and privacy for respondents but also is 'an ethical imperative to establish mutual trust between researchers and narrator' (Kenyon 1996, p.661). Moreover, it 'creates a continuous ethical obligation on the part of the researcher to ensure that the research does not harm the participant and that the privileged position of access...will not be used to the participant's detriment' (Sankar and Gubrium 1994, p.14).

Second, the rights of vulnerable groups in research need to be protected (Kayser-Jones and Koenig 1994; Weaver-Moore and Miller 1999). The complexity and importance of these ethical issues is heightened when research with older people with dementia is considered. While guidance on these matters is limited, the Law Commission report (1993; see Agarwal *et al.* 1996; Lord Chancellor's Department 1997) has some potential application to dementia research. The Law Commission report sets out some important basic principles with respect to 'mentally incapacitated adults' and decision making and recommends that the assessment of whether or not a person lacks the capacity to make a decision needs to include both the nature of the decision and the person's own situation. This suggests, therefore, that there is no uniform approach to involving people with dementia in the decision-making process. Third, the potential risks to participants need to be balanced in relation to possible wider benefits that may result from research.

Berghmans and Ter Meulen (1995) highlight the importance of the ethical principles of beneficence and non-maleficence (doing no harm) in research with dementia patients. They argue that in dementia care research, seldom is there direct benefit to the individual, although the primary aim might be the growth of knowledge and improvement of care in the future. Indeed, by subjecting people with dementia who are unable to decide for themselves about participation in research, the obligation to do good may be put at risk and even infringe the obligation to do no harm to the participant. However, Berghans and Ter Meulen (1995) suggest that the problem can be overcome by making a distinction between therapeutic and non-therapeutic research, where therapeutic research may generally benefit the patient, while non-therapeutic research has no direct benefits for the patient. They conclude that it is illegal or immoral to subject incompetent patients with dementia to research that will not benefit them.

The guidelines proposed by Berghans and Ter Meulen (1995), while helping clarify many important issues, tend to oversimplify a very complex area, and offer little help for researchers tackling the social aspects of dementia care. Other guidelines have recommended a 'common sense' approach to research involving those with conditions such as dementia, especially when advances are most needed and which cannot be obtained by studying other patients or client groups (Royal College of Psychiatrists 1990). Indeed, the Medical Research Council (1991) argues that lack of consent competence should not be grounds for excluding persons suffering from mental incapacity from socially responsible non-therapeutic research, provided safeguards are observed. These include:

> that participation is sought only in research relevant to the individual's condition and where knowledge could not be gained by research with persons able to give consent

> that the research is approved by the appropriate Local Research Ethics Committee (LREC)

> that the participant does not object or appear to object in either words or action

that participation would place the individual at no more than negligible risk of harm and would not be against that individual's best interests.

Many of these questions will be returned to later in this chapter, including the notion of informed consent and future benefits of research.

Involving the person with dementia in the research process

The potential for involving older people with dementia as active subjects in the research process reflects an underlying change in the way dementia is known. As the single, overarching medical model of dementia is increasingly challenged, the possibility of multiple and different understandings of dementia have been uncovered (Clarke 1999; Crossan and McColgan 1999; Harding and Palfrey 1997; Kitwood 1997). This shift in thinking has resulted in changes in the care and research associated with the person with dementia. First, the way that the medicalisation of dementia located the problem with the individual person has been criticised; and now there is greater emphasis on socio-political factors that mediate the experience of dementia. Second, the objectification of the person with dementia has been challenged, and promoting an understanding of their subjective experiences is increasingly desired. Third, the degree to which a person with dementia may be extended the opportunity to be involved in decisions about their everyday life has been questioned. This can range along a continuum from being denied the chance to make decisions in the medical model to their views being fully sought as active partners in their own care (see Clarke 1999 for a summary). Finally, knowledge of subjective experiences that were predominately mediated via the views of family and caregivers has now been widened to include the involvement of the older person with dementia in the research process (Clarke 1999). These important changes have, at the same time, resulted in new and challenging ethical and methodological dilemmas for researchers in dementia care.

Informed consent

The ethical requirement of obtaining informed consent from research participants can be problematic in cases where decision-making capacity is impaired. Not only do procedures to obtain informed consent give rise to feelings of anxiety and insecurity, especially if written consent is required, but questions about the feasibility of actually obtaining informed consent with participants who have dementia are also raised. If a research participant is cognitively impaired, he/she may not understand that he/she is being asked to participate in research. To date, most efforts to deal with ethical issues concerning dementia research have been derived from general ethical principles. Little guidance is available on research involving people with dementia. The Law Commission (1993) sets out guidelines for capacity to consent with treatment, but leaves open the issues of research procedures. In a small study of 15 research participants with early dementia, Agarwal *et al.* (1996) found that no participants fulfilled the Law Commission's criteria for informed consent.

The process of gaining informed consent has been noted to involve three aspects: (1) the person is fully informed; (2) consent is given freely and willingly; and (3) the person is competent (Berghmans and Ter Meulen 1995; Crossan and McColgan 1999). It is evident that any part of this process may be problematic when a person experiences cognitive impairment due to dementia. Whether a person is competent to consent is, probably, the most challenging dilemma and this relates to their ability to be involved in the decision-making process. However, lack of competence cannot be assumed just because a person has a diagnosis of dementia. The level of competency will be determined by the nature of the decision to be made (Kayser-Jones and Koenig 1994; Shah and Dickenson 1999).

The nature of qualitative research also means that the process of consent is not a single event but a continual, on-going process between the researcher and participant (Kayser-Jones and Koenig 1994). This is especially evident when the person may forget that he/she has consented to participate and may require continual reminders. There is the further issue about whether consent needs to be re-negotiated on every visit. Clarification is needed on the issues of consent remaining valid throughout the course of a study, and this is important if the use of advanced directives is to be explored for those in the early stages of dementia.

While arguments have been made for the use of advance directives in dementia research (Bartlett and Martin 2000; Berghmans 1998), this would require researchers to obtain consent from participants in the early stages of their disease, before they become incompetent. However, High (1993) argues that this is practical only in longitudinal studies and not other kinds of study. High further notes that where this has been practised in the USA, researchers also employ an informed consent or assent process when the study commences.

An important issue when considering whether a person is fully informed or not, is whether he/she is aware of his/her diagnosis. Clarke and Keady (1996) found during their study that some of their participants with dementia and their carers did not know about the diagnosis. Even when a medical doctor says a person knows his/her diagnosis, it may have been hidden behind phrases such as 'memory problems' (Crossan and McColgan 1999). This results in major ethical and methodological dilemmas for researchers. For example, how is the study introduced to the participant? Could the respondent feel misled if he/she is unaware that the focus of the study is dementia? Would using the term 'dementia' cause unnecessary harm and distress to the person?

Seeking assent

If the requirement of informed consent were to be applied stringently for all forms of social and medical research, then it would be difficult to justify ethically any research with people suffering from dementia. However, the assent of a representative of the patient may be considered an appropriate alternative when informed consent of the research participant is not possible. The question raised is who is the most appropriate person to give assent? It is assumed that a family member can legitimately step into this role. While this might be logical in the case of urgent clinical interventions, the choice is less clear in dementia research. In research undertaken by Stalker *et al.* (1999a) with people with learning difficulties, the participant's psychiatrist was approached to obtain assent for those judged unable to make an informed decision. Families were not used in the belief that this perpetuated a paternalistic attitude in which those with learning difficulties were regarded as children. The Medical Research Council (1991), on the other hand, points out that the approval of a relative or other independent person is unlikely to be recognised by the law as an adequate substitute for the consent of the research participant, but nevertheless recommends that an independent person is consulted about safeguarding the participant's welfare and interests.

While recognising the various arguments, informed consent is largely a process of communication of information and understanding, and effective family member (or surrogate) participation and cooperation are therefore virtually indispensable. However, there is little practical guidance available on the best way to involve carers. In a study of residents with dementia, Barnett (2000) wrote to relatives first, then talked with residents. She obtained consent verbally then arranged for a 'confidentiality agreement' to be signed between the participant and herself.

Assessment of competency

There are two issues about competency to consider in dementia research. The first is whether it is ethical to undertake research with people who are 'incompetent', and second, how can competency be measured? As with any ethical issue, several opposing views can be identified in the literature. On the one hand, it is argued that 'those kinds of research with incompetent patients, including dementia patients, which do not harm them, and are thus not against their interest are justified, even if patients are unable to give their free consent'. This view is supported by Agarwal *et al.* (1996), who argue that providing research is acting in patients' best interests, and that the study has no side-effects, then unless a patient has actively expressed a desire not to participate it is unlikely to violate fundamental rights. Contradicting this view, however, it is argued that harm is indeed caused if researchers intrude in others' lives without their knowledge, infringing their privacy. Berghmans and Ter Meulen (1995) set out a number of conditions that should be met before non-therapeutic research with incompetent patients with dementia is justified:

1. The research cannot be conducted with a less vulnerable population, e.g. not yet seriously demented and still competent patients or healthy volunteers.

2.   The research must be scientifically sound and promising, with a reasonable expectation of benefit for future patients with dementia.

3.   The research must imply no more than minimal burdens and risks for the patient participant.

4.   The informed consent by a legal representative of the patient must be given (proxy consent). This person should have concern for the values and well-being of the patient.

5.   Researchers should be sensitive to verbal and non-verbal signs and signals that must be interpreted as symptoms of distress resulting from participation in the research project.

The need for a clearer definition of competency and the process by which competency is established by the investigator/person getting the consent has been identified (High 1993). In a large study of care home residents, Fisk and Wigley (2000) developed a screening test that could be used to detect whether residents would be able to give reasoned responses to the interview questions. This screening procedure formed part of the overall interview, so that those that 'passed' went on to complete the remainder of the interview, and for those that did not, the interview was concluded. The focus of the screening procedure was the ability and willingness of those interviewed to:

give answers that were logically related to the question

give answers showing recall of recent events

express an opinion relating to experience of living in their care home

demonstrate a reasonable attention span.

Criteria related to the number of 'don't know' or 'can't remember' answers were established to determine who should continue with the interview. The authors concluded that this procedure was effective 'in maximising the potential for inclusion of residents with cognitive impairments' (Fisk and Wigley 2000, p.32).

Lessons from a study of empowerment

Overview

The purpose of this study, expected to be completed by the end of 2001, is to explore how decisions are made for older people with dementia. That is, to identify the opportunities that exist for people with dementia to be involved in how they live, the barriers to realising these opportunities, and practices that can overcome these barriers. In particular, the aim is to examine how the rights and choices of people with dementia can be balanced with possible concerns that people have for their safety and well-being. Comparisons are to be made between different care settings, namely, residential homes, sheltered housing and the community. The focus of the research is to explore these issues from the perspectives of older people with dementia and their carers in order to understand more about their experiences. For this reason, the research design is qualitative, and includes interviews, participant observation and case studies. The main outcomes of the research will be principles for good practice to promote the empowerment of older people with dementia.

Approval for the study was required from two Local Research Ethics Committees (LRECs) and this was granted following some minor amendments. The study design involved two stages. In stage one 36 individual interviews and 8 focus groups were involved with non-cognitively impaired older people in different settings, care staff, and family members. The data from this stage provides a framework for the next stage, which focuses on older people with dementia in the different settings. The second stage involves interviews with 18 older people with dementia to map decision-making pathways. This includes analysis of case records, and interviews with health professionals, family members and carers. Six case studies will be selected for further in-depth investigation, including participant observation, to explore decision-making in practice, identifying factors that facilitate and hinder empowerment.

Issues in negotiating gatekeepers

In the early months of the project, considerable time was spent in exploring the ethical issues and developing a proposal to safeguard the participants. As the process of negotiating access to older people with dementia commenced, we soon became aware of the multiple layers of protection that surround this group of people. Before approaching potential participants to see if they would be interested in being involved in the study, a number of procedures and gatekeepers had to be negotiated, including: (1) LRECs; (2) levels of senior and middle management; (3) health professionals and/or service providers; and (4) family members. The access to participants was influenced to a great extent by the various gatekeepers' views about involving older people with dementia in research. The study design therefore accommodated these external preferences in a number of ways.

First, in the early stages of proposal development the use of a tool to assess the levels of memory and orientation of participants was considered. This would help determine whether these factors had an effect on their decision-making opportunities. A range of such tools considered included the Mini Mental State Examination (MMSE). However, a gatekeeper, at a senior level, requested that no tool for assessing the cognitive level of the participants be administered directly. While some of the limitations of tools such as the MMSE have been documented (Fisk and Wigley 2000; Stalker *et al.* 1999b), the opportunity to assess the advantages and disadvantages of any tool with people with dementia was removed from the researchers, otherwise access to participants would have been denied. To overcome this problem, it was decided to use the Behavioural Assessment Scale of Later Life (BASOLL) (Brooker 1997a, 1997b; Brooker *et al.* 1993), which assesses the level of self-care, memory, orientation and perceived challenging behaviour of people with dementia. BASOLL is administered to either a staff member or relative in order to assess the capacity of the participant to provide personal informed consent.

Second, the LRECs requested that written assent from a family member be obtained. Whilst this procedure may be considered an important layer of protection to ensure the rights of a vulnerable population, assent may also be considered as disempowering to a person who has made their own decisions throughout their life (Crossan and McColgan 1999). A further dilemma faced by the research team was that of identifying the appropriate family member and/or significant other, and how to involve him/her in the decision-making process. Assent was clearly problematic in the absence of any relatives or significant other, or where the only relative lived overseas and had little or no contact with the potential participant. In such cases, and in the absence of a legal guardian, the home manager took on the role of advocate and provided assent. When someone within the family was identified, the researchers needed to decide whether to approach the potential participant or their family member first. It was decided that there was no uniform approach to this dilemma, and the choice would depend on the individual circumstances of each potential participant. In this way the heterogeneous and complex nature of the participants' social worlds was reflected.

Third, discrepancies existed between the criteria that different LRECs designated in order for the project to gain ethical approval. For example, one LREC requested that a gatekeeper (either a warden or residential home manager) identified and approached potential participants to gain their initial consent. As a consequence of this procedure there was a danger that the sampling was dependent on how the gatekeeper perceived the research, the type of relationship he/she had with his/her residents/tenants, and his/her own judgements on who may be considered competent or not to be involved. To reduce the potential for sample bias, the researchers needed to negotiate carefully with the home manager, or other gatekeeper, ensuring that he/she understood the objectives of the study and the need to have an unbiased sample. It was important to be aware of the unequal power relationships that sometimes exist between home managers and their residents, and the potential for coercion, in particular the possible influence on participants to make their own decisions about being involved in the research.

Fourth, in negotiating access, it was interesting to find that certain requests made in relation to the residents with dementia had not been raised in the earlier stage of the study involving non-cognitively impaired residents. For example, in the pilot study, one gatekeeper wished to sit in on interviews because she felt her presence would be reassuring and help the participant feel less threatened. Another gatekeeper wished to establish the family members' cooperation first, believing that relatives would find this more appropriate than dealing directly with the researchers. It was apparent in many cases that a customer relationship existed between care home or day care managers and family members. Sensitive negotiation was required on the part of the researchers to facilitate access to the required range of participants, whilst ensuring that the decision-making capacity of the person with dementia was not overlooked.

During the early stages of the project, it became evident that the central issues of interest, empowerment and involving older people with dementia in the decision-making process, were mirrored in the research process. In order to gain ethical approval for the study it was necessary to consider the underlying tension between the opposing notions of 'empowerment' and 'risk'. Whilst the opportunity to be involved in an interview may be experienced as empowering for the participant, it is imperative that the rights and privacy of people with dementia are safeguarded (Kayser-Jones and Koenig 1994; Stalker *et al.* 1999b).

Accessing participants and gaining consent

Taking into account the requirements of gatekeepers and ethics committees, the sample selection procedure adopted involved the home manager and/or health care professional approaching potential participants, and an identified family member, to establish their interest in participating in the study. A letter of invitation, accompanied by an information pamphlet, was then sent to potential participants and their identified family member. The researchers subsequently arranged to speak with potential participants about the study and gain their informed consent where possible. The project was explained in a sensitive and unhurried manner, allowing the participant plenty of time to ask questions. This meeting also served as an exploratory interview to establish the level of competence to participate in the research. Assent from the family member/carer was also obtained where available. This practice of 'double consents' was identified by High (1993) in a study of 99 Alzheimer disease projects in the USA. Given the number of interested parties, the sample selection phase took several weeks before it was completed.

To assist the participants' understanding, the information leaflet was developed with very simple and clear information about the study and researchers (see also Dementia Services Development Centre 1996). This was reviewed by clinicians and researchers with experience in the field of dementia, and piloted with a small number of people with dementia.

One of the problems encountered in presenting information about the study was the use of the term 'dementia'. After considerable debate among the research team and advisory group, the term 'memory problems' was used rather than 'dementia' when introducing the project and in questioning the person's own understanding. While it could be argued that, ethically speaking, this was a form of deception, there was the need to balance this issue with the ethical obligation to minimise any potential distress and/or harm to participants. Furthermore, there was a need to work within the limitations of a society that still stigmatises dementia, and in a situation where many individuals were unaware of their diagnoses. However, the ethical dilemmas that surround this issue remain, and researchers need to be explicit about how they approach this issue.

Conclusion

The aim of this chapter has been to analyse critically some of the complex issues challenging dementia research and offer more insight into how such issues can be addressed through experiences gained from a project on empowerment of older people with dementia. Many complex ethical and methodological dilemmas were tackled in this study. How can the person with dementia be involved in the decision-making process associated with informed consent? Whose voices predominate in the multiple layers of protection that surround the person with dementia? How can the opportunity for people to be involved in research be balanced with an ethical obligation not to cause harm to participants? It is evident when considering these questions that issues related to knowledge and power are important aspects of the research process, just as they are in the provision of dementia care.

A central aim of the study reported above is to hear the voices of older people with dementia and to ensure their active participation in the research. Given the fairly recent shift in thinking about researching people with dementia, the available experience from which to develop principles of ethical dementia research practice is still quite limited. This perhaps explains why the published dementia research literature often lacks clarity in relation to ethical issues such as informed consent or why data collection procedures are not made explicit. While the preparation of definitive guidelines is clearly difficult in this complex area of research, there is need to build good practice that can assist ethics committees, gatekeepers and researchers to ensure that empowerment and risk can be appropriately balanced for people with dementia who participate in research.

Note

1   The study is a collaboration between the Oxford Dementia Centre and Anchor Trust, funded by the Community Fund.

References

Adams, T. and Clarke, C. (eds) (1999) *Dementia Care. Developing Partnerships in Practice.* London: Bailliere Tindall.

Agarwal, M., Ferran, J., Ost, K. and Wilson, K. (1996) 'Ethics of "informed consent" in dementia research – the debate continues.' *International Journal of Geriatric Psychiatry 11*, 801–806.

Barnett, E. (2000) *Including the Person with Dementia in Designing and Delivering Care.* London: Jessica Kingsley Publishers.

Bartlett, H. and Martin, W. (2000) 'A balancing act.' *Society Guardian,* p.127, 6 September.

Baskin, S., Morris, J., Ahronheim, J., Meier, D. and Morrison, R. (1998) 'Barriers to obtaining consent in dementia research: Implications for surrogate decision-making.' *Journal of the American Geriatrics Society 46*, 287–290.

Berghmans, R. (1998) 'Advance directives for non-therapeutic dementia research: Some ethical and policy considerations.' *Journal of Medical Ethics 24*, 32–37.

Berghmans, R. and Ter Meulen, R. (1995) 'Ethical issues in research with dementia patients' *International Journal of Geriatric Psychiatry 10*, 647–651.

Bond, J., and Corner, L. (2001) 'Researching dementia: Are there unique methodological challenges for health services research?' *Ageing and Society 21*, 95–116.

Brooker, D. (1997a) *BASOLL: The behavioural assessment scale of later life. Interview form.* Bicester: Winslow Press.

Brooker, D. (1997b) *BASOLL: The behavioural assessment scale of later life. Checklist form.* Bicester: Winslow Press.

Brooker, D., Sturmey, P., Gatherer, A., and Summerbell, C. (1993) 'The behavioural assessment scale of later life (BASOLL): A description, factor analysis, scale development, validity and reliability data for a new scale for older adults.' *International Journal of Geriatric Psychiatry 8*, 747–754.

Clarke, C. (1999) 'Dementia care partnerships: knowledge, ownership and exchange.' In T. Adams and C. Clarke (eds) *Dementia Care. Developing Partnerships in Practice,* pp.5–36. London: Baillière Tindall.

Clarke, C. and Keady, J. (1996) 'Researching dementia care and family caregiving: Extending ethical responsibilities.' *Health Care in Later Life 1*, 2, 85–95.

Crossan, B. and McColgan, G. (1999) 'Informed consent: Old issues re-examined with reference to research involving people with dementia.' Paper (unpublished) presented at British Sociological Association Annual Conference, University of Glasgow.

Dementia Services Development Centre (1996) 'Hearing the voice of people with dementia.' *Green Leaflet Series*. University of Stirling.

Downs, M. (1997) 'The emergence of the person in dementia research.' *Ageing and Society 17*, 597–607.

Fisk, M. and Wigley, V. (2000) 'Accessing and interviewing the oldest old in care homes.' *Quality in Ageing – Policy, Practice and Research 1*, 1, 27–33.

Goldsmith, M. (1996) *Hearing the voice of people with dementia: Opportunities and Obstacles.* London: Jessica Kingsley Publishers.

Harding, N. and Palfrey, C. (1997) *The Social Construction of Dementia: Confused Professionals?* London: Jessica Kingsley Publishers.

High, D. (1993) 'Advancing research with Alzheimer disease subjects: Investigators' perceptions and ethical issues.' *Alzheimer Disease and Associated Disorders 7*, 3, 165–178.

Kayser-Jones, J. and Koenig, B. (1994) 'Ethical issues.' In J. Gubrium and A. Sankar (eds) *Qualitative Methods in Aging Research*, pp.15–32. London: Sage.

Kenyon, G. (1996) 'Ethical issues in ageing and biography.' *Ageing and Society 16*, 659–675.

Kitwood, T. (1997) *Dementia Reconsidered. The Person Comes First.* Buckingham: Open University Press.

Law Commission (1993) *Mentally Incapacitated Adults and Decision-making: Medical treatment and research.* Consultation Paper No.129. London: HMSO.

Lord Chancellor's Department (1997) *Who decides? Making Decisions on Behalf of Mentally Incapacitated Adults.* Cm 3803. London: The Stationery Office.

Medical Research Council (1991) *The Ethical Conduct of Research on the Mentally Incapacitated.* London: MRC.

Royal College of Psychiatrists (1990) *Guidelines for Ethics of Research Committees in Medical Research Involving Human Subjects.* London: RCPsych.

Sankar, A. and Gubrium, J. (1994) 'Introduction.' In J. Gubrium and A. Sankar (eds) *Qualitative Methods in Aging Research*, pp.vii–xvii. London: Sage.

Shah, A. and Dickenson, D. (1999) 'The capacity to make decisions in dementia: some contemporary issues.' *International Journal of Geriatric Psychiatry 14*, 803–806.

Stalker, K., Duckett, P. and Downs, M. (1999a) *Going with the Flow: Choice, Dementia and People with Learning Difficulties.* Brighton: Pavillion.

Stalker, K., Gilliard, J. and Downs, M. (1999b) 'Eliciting user perspectives on what works.' *International Journal of Geriatric Psychiatry 14*, 120–134.

Weaver-Moore, L. and Miller, M. (1999) 'Initiating research with doubly vulnerable populations.' *Journal of Advanced Nursing 30*, 5, 1034–1040.

Chapter Four

Including the perspectives of older people in institutional care during the consent process

Gill Hubbard, Murna Downs and Susan Tester

Introduction

Since the 1980s, there has been a burgeoning commitment to develop understandings of quality of life and quality of care by directly exploring the perspectives and subjective experiences of older people in institutional care settings, many of whom will have dementia (Barnes and Bennett 1998; Browne, McGee and O'Boyle 1997a, 1997b; Coen *et al.* 1993; Forbes 1996; Gubrium 1993, 1995; Mitchell and Koch 1997; Raynes 1998; Spalding and Frank 1985; Splann Krothe 1997). This relatively new concern has led to researchers exploring ways in which they can actively place older people at the heart of the research endeavour and listen to their voice throughout each stage of the investigation (Reed and Payton 1996). The consent procedure is one stage of the research process where there is considerable discussion over the extent to which it is possible for the voice of the older person in institutional care to be heard.

Research ethics require that each person who is participating in the investigation give 'informed consent'. Within medical and social research discourses, informed consent has the same meaning, that is: (1) the person being asked to consent is competent; (2) consent is voluntary and free from coercion; (3) research participants are fully informed about the aims of the research and the consequences of both participating and not participating (American Geriatrics Society 1998; British Sociological Association 2001). Informed consent is a principle that remains a 'central canon of medical research' (Berghmans and Ter Meulen 1995, p.648) and is regarded as a 'cornerstone of protection of human participants in research' (Sachs *et al.* 1994, p.403).

There are, at least, three aspects to consider regarding the issue of consent with older people in institutional care settings. These are: (1) assessment of a person's ability to give informed consent; (2) consent strategies for a person who is deemed unable to give informed consent; and (3) consent strategies for a person who is able to give informed consent. The aim of this chapter is to use this conceptualisation of consent to analyse our own experiences of researching older people in institutional care settings rather than providing an exhaustive review of these three main aspects. Our study is an exploration of the perceptions of quality of life of frail older people in institutional care settings in Scotland and includes older people with physical, sensory and/or cognitive impairments.

Assessment

There has been discussion about the issue of consent within the dementia research literature which has focused on the assessment of a person's ability to give informed consent (Agarwal *et al.* 1996; American Geriatrics Society 1998; Appelbaum and Grisso 1988; Berghmans and Ter Meulen 1995; Helmchen 1990; Kitwood 1995; Marson *et al.* 1994; Sachs *et al.* 1994; Shah, Foli and Odutoy 1999; Sugarman, McCrory and Hubal 1998). A diagnosis of dementia does not in and of itself mean that a person is incapable of giving informed consent (Marson *et al.* 1994), and physicians frequently disagree in their competency judgements (Marson *et al.* 1994). However, it is well accepted that during the onset and progression of dementia, difficulties in comprehending, making judgements, reasoning, communicating and remembering may limit the scope of a person's decision-making capabilities.

One of the points that this literature has raised is that a person's ability to make a decision about whether to participate in research may periodically vary because the ways in which dementia affects a person's cognitive abilities are not static but fluctuate. Marson *et al.* (1994, p.9) describe fluctuations in decision-making capacity as 'intermittent competency' and propose that researchers devise periodic evaluations of competency. In this sense, the ability to give informed consent is viewed as an on-going process and, as such, researchers need to assess continuously a person's decision-making capacity to find out if he/she is able to provide informed consent to participate in research.

The literature also highlights the need to assess a person's ability to give informed consent in the context of what the person is being asked to do (American Geriatrics Society 1998; Marson *et al.* 1994). The American Geriatrics Society (1998, p.1308) recommend that, 'The capacity to obtain informed consent should be assessed in each individual for each research protocol being considered'. Although a person with dementia may not be competent to make a decision about one particular research project he/she may be able to make a competent decision with respect to other research initiatives. This notion of task-specific consent may be applied to the different tasks *within* a particular research project. For example, a person may be deemed competent to decide whether to be included in the general observations of the nursing home but may not be competent to decide whether or not to be included in an aspect of the investigation which will involve him/her being video-recorded. Asking older people who may be unfamiliar with latest technologies to give their informed consent to have their interview transcripts stored within a data archive such as Economic and Social Research Council Qualidata, and to consent to have their research findings published on the web, may be particularly problematic.

Strategies

There has also been some discussion about how researchers should proceed when someone with a cognitive impairment has been deemed unable to give informed consent. A number of solutions have been proposed including surrogate decision-making (Baskin *et al.* 1998; Dukoff and Sunderland 1997; Sachs *et al.* 1994) and advance consent directives

(Dukoff and Sunderland 1997; Sachs 1994). However, these solutions are not without their own difficulties. For instance, one of the problems with advance consent directives is that there may be a time lapse between making a decision about whether or not to participate in research and a research project taking place. Sachs (1994, p.24) uses this point to criticise 'formal advance consent directives' because they may occur some time, possibly years, before research actually begins. He believes that, 'Clearly, one normally feels more confident acting upon a patient's or subject's prior statements when those statements have been made recently and when they specifically address the decision at hand' (p.24). This is why he recommends that researchers and health care professionals view advance consent directives as a 'process' rather than as an 'event'.

Although proxy consent is often sought, there is a general acceptance that relying exclusively on proxy consent, whilst ostensibly meeting ethical guidelines, may not be a fully ethical way to conduct research. For this reason various procedures have been suggested for use in conjunction with proxy consent. For instance, researchers could find out about a person's own willingness to take part in an investigation *before* the research takes place. It has been found that even those people identified as unable to give informed consent to participate in research are still able to supply information about their values and preferences which can be used by researchers when deciding whether to include them in the research (Sachs *et al.* 1994). Another suggestion is that researchers be vigilant and continue to seek a person's willingness to take part in an investigation *during* the research process. Berghmans and Ter Meulen (1995, p.651) recommend that researchers need to be 'very sensitive to verbal and non-verbal signs and signals' so that if a participant shows symptoms of distress then they should be immediately withdrawn from the investigation. Using this approach, researchers are able to use 'behavioural consent' to monitor continuously a person's willingness to consent to be included in the research. Other researchers have also advocated a strategy of negotiated consent whereby researchers continuously assess a participant's willingness to remain included in the investigation (Reed and Payton 1996).

These consent strategies for people who are deemed unable to give informed consent are reflected in recent legislation. The Adults with Incapacity (Scotland) Act 2000 clearly specifies that in cases where a person is deemed unable to give informed consent to participate in research, then this consent has to be obtained from a guardian, welfare attorney or relative. The Act encourages people to designate a surrogate decision maker before they lose their ability to give informed consent. The Act also specifies that the incapacitated adult must be willing to participate in the research and that, 'the present and past wishes and feelings of the adult so far as they can be ascertained by any means of communication, whether human or by mechanical aid (whether of an interpretative nature or otherwise) appropriate to the adult' (HMSO 2000) must be taken into account. This implies that researchers will need to assess continuously whether people who are incapacitated still wish to be involved in the investigation and continuously monitor whether or not they are distressed. The concept of continuous consent is reinforced by the fifth principle of the Act which stresses that adults who are incapacitated must be encouraged 'to exercise whatever skills' and to 'develop new skills' so that they are able to take some control over their lives. This suggests that people who are deemed unable to give informed consent should be encouraged to make decisions continuously about their role in the research process even if their consent to participate is by proxy (HMSO 2000).

Strategies that have been recommended for people who are deemed unable to give informed consent are also applicable to those who are able to give informed consent. It is generally accepted that people who have given informed consent before the research takes place ought to be able to withdraw from the investigation at any time. One of the difficulties that has been found in researching frail older people in institutional care settings who have given informed consent, however, is that some of them may not consistently remember what the research project is about and what they have consented to. A solution that has been used with people who have difficulties remembering is to remind them continuously of what the project is about each time that the researcher visits the facility (Crossan and McColgan 1999).

While there may be a general acceptance that researchers continually ascertain the willingness of participants to remain involved in the investigation, this principle is yet to be explicitly stated in many of the ethical guidelines. There are a range of professional societies that could usefully provide ethical guidelines for researchers working with older people in institutional care settings. For example, the American Geriatrics Society and the British Society of Gerontology by definition focus on research of older people. However, a number of researchers working in this field may also reference societies within their own subject disciplines such as the British Sociological Association and the British Psychological Society for ethical guidance. To date, the British Society of Gerontology provide no ethical guidelines, whilst the American Geriatrics Society in 1998 issued a position statement on 'Informed consent for research on human subjects with dementia'. The British Sociological Association (2001) present ethical guidelines that also emphasise the concept of informed consent. The Association recommend that, 'As far as possible sociological research should be based on the freely given informed consent of those studied'. It also advises that, 'where research participants are ill or too young or too old to participate, proxies may need to be used in order to gather data'. Whilst these ethical guidelines highlight the importance of the principle of informed consent, they have yet to embrace the critical mass, which is recognising that there needs to be a variety of strategies for continuously ascertaining the willingness of a person to engage in research, whether they have given informed consent, an advance consent directive, or proxy consent.

Despite the complexities involved in gaining consent, few researchers have described this process in any detail. Most of the existing literature is theoretical rather than grounded in the actual experience of obtaining consent. This chapter describes the ways in which we as researchers practically obtained the consent of research participants. In the process of reflecting upon our own research practice we analyse the extent to which implementing consent as a process rather than an a priori event provides more opportunities for listening to the perspectives of older people in institutional care in research. Further progress can be made on this complex ethical terrain if there is a move away from abstract generalities and a move towards concrete, practical situations becoming 'much more empirical' and attending to the 'content of research but also to the process' (Kitwood 1995, p.657).

Gathering consent during our research

The aim of the research on which this chapter is based is to explore the perceptions of quality of life of frail older people in institutional care settings in Scotland. Existing work on older people's perspectives has tended to exclude those in institutional care with the most severe disabilities and with whom communication is most difficult as a result of sensory and cognitive impairment(s) (Farquhar 1995). We wanted to include all older people in our research, including those who are unable to give informed consent. The study involves two phases of data collection in the institutional care settings which were nursing and residential homes: (1) general observations in the institutions; (2) being with, and conversing with individual residents who have recently entered the institution. In the following sections we reflect upon our own experiences of gaining ethical approval, assessing competency, and gathering consent for the first phase.

Two health board ethics committees and one social work department were approached for ethical approval for our research. We outlined in detail on the ethical approval applications our consent procedure. With reference to carrying out the general observations in the nursing/residential homes we stated that we would seek informed consent from the residents, relatives and nursing home staff. If the resident was unable to give informed consent relatives would be informed about the study and asked to sign a consent form giving permission to include their relative in the study. The ethics committees and social work department approved of our research on an understanding that consent was gathered before the research commenced. They were also satisfied that those residents identified as unable to give informed consent would consent by proxy.

We now reflect upon our own research practices and the ways in which we gathered the consent of older people for carrying out the general observations in institutional care. There were two key stages to the consent process: (1) gathering informed consent or proxy consent *before* the research took place, and (2) gathering consent *during* the research process.

Once access to residents in nursing and residential homes was made possible by gaining approval of the research project from the relevant ethics committees and social work department we were required to gain proxy consent for those residents who were unable to give informed consent. Therefore, we needed some way of assessing whether or not the older person was competent. Our solution was to ask the nursing or residential home manager to decide which of her residents she believed were able to give informed consent. The manager was asked to base her decision on a resident's ability to understand the aims of the research and what participation in the research would involve.

The residents who were designated by the manager as able to give informed consent were directly approached by the researchers and asked if they would agree to become involved in the investigation. These residents' relatives were not informed that research was taking place in the home, as the researchers felt that this could erode the older person's autonomy and contribute towards a process of infantalisation (Hockey and James 1993). A researcher sat with the resident and explained the aims of the research. The resident was also informed that the identity of the home, the names of the residents who participated in the research, and the information gathered would be kept confidential. An information sheet in large print providing written details about the project was handed to the resident. The resident was asked to sign the consent form that was handed out at the same time. The consent form had a series of questions that were designed to indicate that the resident understood the aims of the research, understood that he or she could withdraw from the research at any time, and that he or she agreed to participate in the investigation. The resident would answer each question with a yes or no response and would only be co-opted into the study if he/she answered affirmatively.

Some residents did not take the information sheet because they said that they could not read it. Others did not sign the consent form either because they could not see to sign their name, found it physically difficult to hold a pen and write, or did not like the idea of having to sign an official-looking form. We took account of sensory and physical impairments and the attitudes of some residents towards signing official forms by enabling these residents to give their consent verbally to participate in the research. This approach was similar to the one adopted by Reed and Payton (1996) who also discovered that not all residents were willing or able to sign a consent form. By using this flexible and sensitive approach we adapted the consent procedure approved of by the ethics committees and social work department which assumed that consent forms would be signed.

The manager of the home had given the researchers a list of residents whom she believed were unable to give informed consent. The relatives of these residents were contacted in writing by the researchers and asked for permission to include their relative in the investigation. An information sheet and consent form similar to those given to the residents who were able to give informed consent were sent to each relative. In one particular home a small number of residents did not have an immediate relative to contact, so the manager made the decision on the resident's behalf instead. Interestingly, the manager did not base her decision on any medical prognosis by excluding those residents with the most severe diagnosis of dementia. Instead, she agreed to include in the research the residents whom she felt would enjoy the experience of participating and excluded those who she believed would become upset and/or angry. This suggests that she focused on residents' emotional dispositions rather than on their cognitive and functional abilities.

One of the major dilemmas facing us was ensuring that the perspectives of all residents, including those who were perceived as unable to give informed consent, were taken into account during the consent procedure. To ensure that all residents, including those with comprehension, memory and communication difficulties, were involved in the consent process we adopted a strategy of on-going consent. Each time that the researchers spent time with a particular resident who had either directly given informed consent or had been co-opted into the investigation by proxy, we explained our presence. We observed this resident's non-verbal behaviours as well as his or her verbal utterances to determine whether the resident wanted to participate in the research at that particular point in time. We provided opportunities for the resident to continuously make sense of the research experience and ask questions about the research. We sat down next to the resident with a notebook in hand and started to observe and make notes. At the same time, we explained our presence and asked if the resident minded if the researcher sat and watched what the resident was doing and chatted to him or her about what she was observing.

Case Examples

The following accounts are descriptions of the ways in which the researchers continued to gather consent during the research process and the ways in which the residents interpreted the research experience. The information in brackets references the nursing home, date of the observation and text lines as stored in the qualitative data software package NUD*IST (Qualitative Solutions and Research 1997). All of the residents who actually declined to participate in the study were asked for consent to have their experiences included in this chapter. The researcher visited each resident and asked their permission to include their experiences. All but one of these residents either verbally or in writing, gave this permission.

Joanne was a resident in one home who clearly indicated that she did not wish to be involved in the investigation on one occasion that the researcher visited the home. This is despite the fact that Joanne had previously given permission to be included in the study and had signed a consent form. As the researcher walked into the lounge, Joanne started to look quickly around the room. Joanne was sitting on one of the settees and as the researcher went over she waved her hand as if to 'shoo' the researcher away and said very sternly 'no comment'. Joanne then got up and with the support of her zimmer-frame left the room (B2 17th November text 12–17).

Susan was another resident who had previously given her consent who clearly indicated through her non-verbal behaviour that she did not wish to participate in the research on one particular day that the researcher visited. Susan was sitting in a chair outside of the lift on the second floor. The researcher sat down in a chair next to her. Susan got up and went to the toilet and when she returned she put her hand up to her forehead, partially hiding her face (B2 26th November text 235–242).

One resident, Rebecca, who had given her consent to participate in the research, even changed her mind about whether to engage with the researcher during one observation session. When the researcher entered the lounge Rebecca said loudly to the researcher, 'Go to your bed.' When a carer brought a chair for the researcher to sit on Rebecca said sternly, 'Take that away, don't sit near me' (D4 14th March text 11). Later, when the researcher was about to leave the lounge, Rebecca asked the researcher,

'What do you say about me?' 'What shall I say about you?' the researcher replied. Rebecca responded, 'That they took away my pension. I've nothing left. Can you do anything about that?' (D4 14th March text 426–428).

These incidents show that some residents make it clear that they do not wish to participate in the research. They also show that residents opt in and out of the investigation, sometimes during the same day. Rebecca's conversation with the researcher suggests that she had a misperception of the role of the researcher. Her question indicates that she had expectations that the researcher was there to sort out particular problems for the residents in the home. A resident in another home who had given informed consent also had similar misperceptions of the role of the researcher. This misperception led him to opt out of the investigation. The researcher sat down next to Arthur and reminded him who she was. He immediately started to talk about why he wanted to return to his own home in the community:

Arthur:	I want out. I want my own home.
Researcher:	Why don't you like it here?
Arthur:	I prefer my own wee house.
Researcher:	Why?
Arthur:	Because it's better than this.
Researcher:	Why?
Arthur:	You wouldn't like to lose you own home would you? (Pause). Because it's better than this. It's terrible. It's like prison. Get me out.
Researcher:	I can't get you out.
Arthur:	You're no use to me then.

(B2 17th November text 20–35)

However, not all residents felt confident about refusing to participate whilst the researcher was present. Instead, they voiced their concerns later and to other people. On one occasion a couple of residents informed their professional care staff after the observation had taken place that they were not happy with the presence of a researcher in the dining room. The carers relayed this information to the researcher and suggested that the residents were unhappy because they did not understand what the research was about, even though they had given their consent on a previous occasion. The researcher sat with the two residents and explained the nature of the research. The two residents appeared satisfied and as the researcher was leaving and walking down the stairs she heard one of them say to the other, 'That's Stirling University' (B2 28th November text 300–358). This example suggests that other people besides the researchers have a role to play and are likely to become involved in the consent process.

It is worth pointing out that all of these examples are residents who were able to give informed consent to participate in the research. None of the residents who were identified as incapable of giving informed consent indicated to the researchers that they did not want to participate. This suggests that researchers need to be more vigilant in recognising when older people who cannot give informed consent do not want to participate in the research.

However, even the residents who were deemed unable to give informed consent clearly understood something about the investigation. Their understandings are reflected in their expressions of curiosity about what the researcher was doing. With the researcher actually sitting with a notepad and making notes, the data collection process became more transparent. Residents, including those deemed unable to give informed consent, showed awareness that the research was taking place and took opportunities to probe the researcher about what she was doing. 'What's that for?' asked one resident whilst pointing to the notepad (C3 12th January text 46–48). 'What are you writing down?' asked another (C3 12th January text 218–219). 'You're a quick writer' observed one resident and later on asked, 'What's it for?' (C3 11th January text 26–52). 'What is it you're doing?' asked one resident (C3 11th January text 321–322). 'Are you left-handed?' asked another resident, whilst observing the researcher making notes (C3 24th January text 55). 'I can't read but it's nice' a resident remarked (C3 24th January text 238–239). When the researcher explained what the investigation was about, one resident responded, 'You'll never find out because people don't tell the truth' (C3 24th January text 65–68).

Although residents may not be able to understand all aspects of the research, they at least understand some. One resident's husband, who also resided in the nursing home, decided on her behalf that she could participate in the study. On one occasion that the researcher visited the home the resident asked the researcher several times how long she had been working at the hospital. Her husband corrected her by saying, 'No, she's from the university' (A1, 23rd October text 103–105). However, on the next day that the researcher visited the home she indicated that she was aware of the next stage of the research when she asked the researcher who was just about to leave, 'Are you going to type it (the fieldnotes) up?' (A1 24th October text 174–175). One reason why some residents' understandings of the research may be partial is because they have difficulties remembering. Even those residents who were perceived by the manager of the nursing/residential home as being able to give informed consent may have experienced difficulties remembering what the research was about. For example, one of Henry's relatives was present during a time that the researcher visited the home. The relative introduced himself to the researcher and pointed out to Henry that the researcher was 'observing'. Henry commented that he had seen the researcher in the home on previous occasions. His relative informed the researcher that Henry remembered people but he would not necessarily recall when it was that he had seen them (A1 12th November 111–146). These two examples show that residents may understand and retain knowledge about some aspects of the research and not others. They also highlight that researchers should not automatically assume that just because a resident is able to give informed consent that they do not need to be reminded about the research.

Some residents developed their understandings of the nature of the investigation and negotiated with the researcher their respective roles within the research endeavour. The two examples described here are both of residents whose consent was by proxy. Jenny appeared to place the researcher in the role of a teacher. The researcher followed Jenny as she walked along the corridor. Jenny asked, 'Are you the teacher coming to teach us?' The researcher said that she was not the teacher to which Jenny replied, 'That's all right' (A1 11th November 87–88). On another occasion that the researcher visited the home Jenny again indicated her understanding of the role of the researcher. 'Are you top of the form?' she asked. 'Can you tell?' replied the researcher. 'Yes' said Jenny (A1 3rd November text 236–248). Other residents placed the researcher in the role of a friend and a companion for the day. 'Have you met my friend?' asked Roseanne, referring to the researcher (C3 11th January text 386). Roseanne liked to wander around the home looking for people to cuddle and chat with and she asked the researcher to accompany her. Her conversation with the researcher highlights that it is not clear whether she wanted the researcher to come with her because she was a 'friend' or because she understood that the researcher was observing and making notes about her behaviour:

Researcher: Is it OK if I sit with you?

Roseanne: I don't mind, I'm going away soon anyway.

Researcher: Do you like to watch TV?

Roseanne: I don't mind.

Researcher: What other things do you like doing besides watching TV?

Roseanne: I didn't say I like watching TV.

Researcher: What do you like doing?

Roseanne: Nothing (Pause). I think I'll go, are you coming?

Researcher: OK I'll follow you.

Later on:

Roseanne: What is it you're doing?

Researcher: I'm writing that you're sitting in a chair.
(Roseanne nods.)

Roseanne: Is that short hand?

(C3 11th January text 283–298)

Other residents highlighted what they felt about being researched and what role they wanted to play in the process. One resident whose consent was by proxy indicated that he wanted to help the researcher and to be useful. Charlie showed the researcher some pieces of paper that he took out of his pocket:

Charlie:	I like to know you've used it and it's been some use to you.'
	(Charlie watched the researcher make notes in her notepad.)
Researcher:	I'm writing that down what you've said.
Charlie:	I'm just watching to see if I can help you if something goes wrong.

(C3 21st January text 327–355)

This conversation developed to illuminate Charlie's financial predicament in the home. Without any money Charlie felt that all that he had to give the researcher was his name. Charlie read out what he had written on the piece of paper:

Charlie:	50p and 30p. There's my full name Charlie Smith. That's all I've got to give you... I'm ashamed to tell you I can't even find a penny, not a penny.
Researcher:	Would you like to have some money on you?
Charlie:	Yes. 30 or 40 to start with, don't worry I'll give you it back.
Researcher:	30 or 40 pence?
Charlie:	Pounds.

(C3 21st January text 327–355)

The above accounts provide a window into the ways in which the researchers gathered consent during the research process and the ways in which older people, including those deemed unable to give informed consent, interpreted the research experience.

Conclusion

Reflections on our own research practice and analysis of data suggest that researchers can continuously monitor a person's willingness to participate in the investigation and can contribute towards developing the participant's understandings about the research. We have shown that some of our participants did opt in and out of the research. However, most of these were residents who had given informed consent. This suggests that we need to find ways in which older people who are deemed unable to give informed consent can also opt in and out of the research. In particular, we need to watch their non-verbal behaviour to assess whether they are willing participants in the research process. We have shown that other people, including professional care staff and friends and relatives, play a role in the consent process. Our findings show that residents, including those deemed unable to give informed consent, possessed some level of understanding of the research. Residents added to their understandings by probing the researcher about her activities whilst she was conducting the observations and by negotiating their, and the researcher's, role during the research process. Providing opportunities for residents to ask questions about the research thus developed participants' understandings of the investigation in practice.

There is a need to protect vulnerable groups of older people from exploitation by researchers who are keen to pursue their own careers and develop new avenues for increasing knowledge and understanding in their particular field (Kitwood 1995). The rights of an older person who is deemed unable to give informed consent should be protected. This means that while there is a need to gather proxy consent before the research commences, there is also a need to continue to gather consent during the research process.

A model of consent in which consent gathering is conceived as a continuous process rather than an a priori event has the potential to provide opportunities for listening to the perspectives of older people in institutional care, including those deemed unable to give informed consent, for the following reasons. Continuous assessment of a person's willingness to participate in the investigation enables the researcher to withdraw that person if they show signs of distress. Continuously negotiating consent provides opportunities for the older person to change his/her mind and to withdraw from and opt in to the study according to his/her needs, giving the older person some control over the research process. Since many older people in institutional care have dementia and may have 'intermittent competency', a process of on-going consent enables the person during their more lucid moments to vent his/her thoughts and feelings about the research even if he/she has entered the research programme by proxy.

Conceptualising consent as a continuous process rather than an a priori event avoids the problems of a time lapse between gaining consent before the research takes place and actually commencing the research. This is because researchers can regularly verify that a person is still willing to be included in the investigation. Constantly monitoring consent enables the researcher to provide opportunities for the older person to consent to specific stages of the research so that the consent process is task-specific and grounded in a framework of what the person is being specifically asked to do. Gathering consent whilst the research takes place is an experiential approach that gives the older person an opportunity actually to experience what it is like to be a research participant. It is an approach that assumes a person who actually experiences the research is more fully informed, because it gives him/her a taste of what it physically and emotionally feels like to be researched, which means that he/she better placed to decide whether to participate or not.

The development of ethical guidelines for good research practice in institutional care settings for older people would be a welcome step forward. These guidelines would have the potential to contribute to the development of active discussion towards conceptualising consent as a continuous process rather than an a priori event. Ethics committees can play a role by questioning the ways in which researchers provide opportunities for the perspectives of older people, including those deemed unable to give informed consent, to be heard during the research process. At the same time, we would welcome further sharing of empirical work and theoretical developments by researchers within this difficult ethical terrain. It is only in this way that researchers will consent to challenge their own understandings and reflect upon their research practices. In this chapter we have shown that whilst it remains important to take account of a person's capability to give informed consent it is also important to recognise that even those people categorised as unable to give informed consent strive to interpret the research experience and negotiate their role. We have shown how older people can become active rather than passive participants in the research process. In doing so, we illuminate the potential for placing the older person in institutional care at the heart of the research endeavour.

Acknowledgements

This paper is based on research undertaken by Gill Hubbard, Susan Tester and Murna Downs, within the Economic and Social Research Council (ESRC) research programme 'Growing Older: Extending Quality Life' (Award Ref. L480 25 4023). Thanks are due to the managers and staff of the nursing/residential homes in which the fieldwork took place. We are particularly grateful to the older people, who have been given fictitious names to protect their anonymity. We would also like to thank Kate Allan, Research Fellow at Stirling University, for her ideas on the issue of consent within the field of dementia.

References

Agarwal, M., Ferran, J., Ost, K. and Wilson, K. (1996) 'Ethics of "informed consent" in dementia research: The debate continues.' *International Journal of Geriatric Psychiatry 11*, 801–806.

American Geriatrics Society (1998) 'Informed consent for research on human subjects with dementia.' *Journal of the American Geriatrics Society 46*, 1308–1310.

Appelbaum, P. and Grisso, T. (1988) 'Assessing patients' capacities to consent to treatment.' *The New England Journal of Medicine 319*, 25, 1635–1638.

Barnes, M. and Bennett, G. (1998) 'Frail bodies, courageous voices: Older people influencing community care.' *Health and Social Care in the Community 6*, 2, 102–111.

Baskin, S., Morris, J., Ahronheim, J., Meier, D. and Morrison, R. (1998) 'Barriers to obtaining consent in dementia research: Implications for surrogate decision-making.' *The American Geriatrics Society 46*, 287–290.

Berghmans, R. and Ter Meulen, R. (1995) 'Ethical issues in research with dementia patients.' *International Journal of Geriatric Psychiatry 10*, 647–651.

British Sociological Association (2001) *Statement of Ethical Practice* http://www.britsoc.org.uk/about/ethic.htm accessed 3 May 2001.

Browne, J., McGee, H. and O'Boyle, C. (1997a) 'Conceptual approaches to the assessment of quality of life.' *Psychology and Health 12*, 737–751.

Browne, J., O'Boyle, C. and McGee, H. (1997b) 'Development of a direct weighting procedure for quality of life domains.' *Quality of Life Research 6*, 301–309.

Coen, R., O'Mahony, D., O'Boyle, C., Joyce, C., Hiltbrunner, B., Walsh, J. and Coakley, D. (1993) 'Measuring the quality of life of dementia patients using the Schedule for the Evaluation of Individual Quality of Life.' *The Irish Journal of Psychology 14*, 1, 154–163.

Crossan, B. and McColgan, G. (1999) 'Informed consent: Old issues re-examined with reference to research involving people with dementia.' Paper presented at the British Sociological Association Annual Conference, Glasgow.

Dukoff, R. and Sunderland, T. (1997) 'Durable power of attorney and informed consent with Alzheimer's disease patients: A clinical study.' *American Journal of Psychiatry 154*, 8, 1070–1075.

Farquhar, M. (1995) 'Elderly people's definitions of quality of life.' *Social Science and Medicine 41*, 10, 1439–1446.

Forbes, D. (1996) 'Clarification of the constructs of satisfaction and dissatisfaction with home care.' *Public Health Nursing 13*, 6, 377–385.

Gubrium, J. (1993) *Speaking of Life.* New York: Aldine de Gruyter.

Gubrium, J. (1995) 'Voice, context and narrative in aging research.' *Canadian Journal on Aging 14*, S1, 68–81.

Helmchen, H. (1990) 'The unsolved problem of informed consent in dementia research.' *Psychiatria Fennica 21*, 163–173.

HMSO (2000) *Adults with Incapacity (Scotland) Act.* <http://www.scotland-legislation.hmso.gov.uk/legislation/scotland/acts2000/20000004.htm> accessed 3 May 2001.

Hockey, J. and James, A. (1993) *Growing up and growing old: Ageing and Dependency in the Lifecourse.* London: Sage.

Kitwood, T. (1995) 'Exploring the ethics of dementia research: A response to Berghmans and Ter Meulen: A psychosocial perspective.' *International Journal of Geriatric Psychiatry 10*, 655–657.

Marson, D., Schmitt. F., Ingram, K. and Harrell, L. (1994) 'Determining the competency of Alzheimer patients to consent to treatment and research.' *Alzheimer Disease and Associated Disorders 8*, 4, 5–18.

Mitchell, P. and Koch, T. (1997) 'An attempt to give nursing home residents a voice in the quality improvement process: The Challenge of frailty.' *Journal of Clinical Nursing 6*, 453–461.

Qualitative Solutions and Research (1997) *QSR NUD*IST User Guide.* Qualitative Solutions and Research Pty Ltd.

Raynes, N. (1998) 'Involving residents in quality specification.' *Ageing and Society 18*, 65–78.

Reed, J. and Payton, V. (1996) 'Past the age of consent? A discussion of some ethical issues arising in a study involving older people.' *Health Care in Later Life 1*, 1, 52–61.

Sachs, G. (1994) 'Advance consent for dementia research.' *Alzheimer Disease and Associated Disorders 8*, 4, 19–27.

Sachs, G., Stocking, C., Stern, R., Cox, D., Hougham, G. and Sachs, R. (1994) 'Ethical aspects of dementia research: Informed consent and proxy consent.' *Clinical Research 42*, 3, 403–412.

Shah, A., Foli, S. and Odutoye, K. (1999) 'Capacity to consent in dementia and the additional costs of implementing the Bournewood judgement in geriatric psychiatry.' *Aging and Mental Health 3*, 2, 153–157.

Spalding, J. and Frank, W. (1985) 'Quality care from the residents' point of view.' *American Health Care Association Journal* July, 3–7.

Splann Krothe, J. (1997) 'Giving voice to elderly people: community-based long-term care.' *Public Health Nursing 14*, 4, 217–226.

Sugarman, J., McCrory, D. and Hubal, R. (1998) 'Getting meaningful informed consent from older adults: A structured literature review of empirical research.' *Journal of the American Geriatrics Society 46*, 4, 517–524.

Chapter Five

Including people with dementia
Advisory networks and user panels

Lynne Corner

Consumer involvement

Consumer involvement in research is a relatively recent phenomenon (Hanley *et al.* 2000). A consumer is someone who has personal or family experience of the health issue or services being considered, or someone who is a formal representative of a consumer panel, with access to other people's experiences and personal knowledge (Bastian 1994). Consumer involvement is the:

> active involvement of consumers in the research process, rather than the use of consumers as the 'subjects' of research. This involvement might occur in any or all of the processes involved in research – setting the research agenda, commissioning research, undertaking research, interpreting research and disseminating the results of research. (Standing Advisory Group on Consumer Involvement 1998)

Whereas there is a real increase in the involvement of consumers in defining the research agenda, commissioning research and disseminating the results of research, direct involvement in undertaking research is quite limited (Carr-Hill and Dixon 1998).

People with dementia have largely been excluded from all stages of the research process, mainly because of the perceived challenges to verbal communication and understanding. This chapter briefly considers the model of involving people with dementia and their carers in identifying topics, priorities and commissioning research used in Quality Research in Dementia (QRD). The involvement of a small panel of people with dementia and carers in the process of on-going research is then discussed and their role in framing research questions and analysing and interpreting interview data described in detail.

Quality Research in Dementia is the research grants programme for the Alzheimer's Society and was launched in 1999 (http://www.alzheimers.org.uk/). A major focus of QRD is to influence the direction of basic scientific research, care practice, health and social policy and to improve quality of life for people with dementia and their carers. The programme funds and evaluates research and contributes to the search for causes, cure and care for dementia. Research also covers the effectiveness of drugs, therapies and care practices and the health and social impact of dementia or carers or the community at large.

A major part of QRD is the QRD Advisory Network. This consists of 100–150 carers and people with dementia, balanced by a similar number of researchers, scientists, clinicians and other experts. QRD matches its research agenda to the real needs of people with dementia and their carers and actively involves people with dementia and carers in setting priorities for research, selecting proposals for funding, monitoring on-going projects and disseminating the outcomes of research. They are also involved in reviewing grant proposals for funding.

Involving people with dementia in a user panel

A user panel consisting of people with dementia and their carers is being used in the development of a 'toolkit' of methods for assessing quality of life, a project funded by the Alzheimer's Society. The project phases are summarised in Table 5.1.

The purpose of the user panel

The main purpose of establishing the user panel was to explore ways of ensuring that as far as possible the research both began, and continued to remain, grounded in the views of people with dementia and their carers. The aims and objectives of the research had already been set and so the

Table 5.1: Phases of the research project

Literature search and review.

Qualitative interview study involving people with dementia, informal and formal carers, health professionals and people without dementia.

Review and selection of outcome measures for assessing quality of life for people with dementia.

Development of toolkit of outcome measures to assess quality of life for people with dementia.

user panel works within set parameters: this was user involvement, as opposed to user-led research. The project is currently on-going, as is the user panel.

Initially, the purposes of the panel were:

> to ensure that the research focused on and reflected the priorities of older people with dementia and their carers

> to give people with dementia and their carers a voice in the research process

> to advise on practical aspects of the research process, including methods of communicating with people with dementia and question design.

A literature search concluded that older people have been involved in research (Barnes and Bennett 1998; Barnes and Wistow 1992; Beresford and Croft 1993). However, while there were many cases of older people with dementia and their carers being involved as the subjects of research, there were few examples of their involvement in undertaking research (Barnes and Bennett-Emslie 1997). This meant that there were no guidelines as to how a panel might be established, how to involve people or what their role would be. As our starting point we assumed that some older people with dementia and carers would want to be involved, given that there was no evidence to suggest otherwise! We felt strongly however that the perspective of the person with dementia had traditionally been neglected in approaches to examining their quality of life. Also, while the views of people with dementia might be sought in the initial stages of the project, as the data is refined and analysed the original meaning and context of what was said can be blurred. It therefore seemed very important to ensure that people with dementia had a voice on the project team. On the other hand, we had some ambivalence about establishing a user panel. We wondered whether the involvement of people with dementia would merely be 'political correctness' and their contribution 'tokenism', with the research agenda and decision making remaining very much under the control of the researchers.

Establishing the user panel

A series of articles were published in national, regional and local Alzheimer Society newsletters describing the research project and asking people to contact the research team if they wanted any information. The purpose of this was merely to advertise the project's existence, not to recruit people to the user panel. Our original intention was to establish the panel some months later, following a literature review. However, at this stage three people wrote expressing an interest in the project and volunteering to take part as research subjects. The main requirement of the panel was that people were interested in and motivated by the project and so, although the qualitative study was not due to start for some months, we made a pragmatic decision to take the opportunity to start the user panel earlier than planned. We contacted the people who had volunteered with a view to them becoming part of the user panel. A researcher visited each person and explained the aims and objectives of the research and raised the idea of a user panel. The three (one person with dementia, two carers) were enthusiastic about taking part in the project, although they were initially unclear what their role might be and unsure whether they would have anything useful to offer. A further two people were identified through subsequent visits to local Alzheimer Societies and a member of the local Alzheimer Society also agreed to join.

The panel consists of four women and three men, who either have dementia or are informal or formal carers, a professional from the local branch of the Alzheimer's Society, and the author. Three people have dementia and two are carers. The age range is 62–83 years old. There are two married couples, and one person with dementia who lives alone. The three members who have dementia have been diagnosed for nine months, four years and eight years respectively, and have mild or moderate dementia. They are all retired, but are from different backgrounds and live in different parts of the study area.

The project is funded for three years and the members of the user panel were asked to commit for six months in the first instance, but with a view to taking part in the whole project. Consent is formally reviewed on a three-monthly basis, and members know that they are free to leave the panel at any time. To help the panel understand the aims and objectives of the research and their proposed role in the research team, an information pack was prepared. 'Informed consent' was an important issue and its meaning in this setting needed much consideration. It was difficult to know what and how much information to give to panel members to ensure they were able to make an informed decision about whether to take part. The pack included a lay summary of the proposal, a simple glossary of research terms and techniques, and issues of confidentiality and anonymity. The amount of information required by different panel members varied both in terms of the quantity and times when they required it.

The form of the user panel

A deliberate decision was made to keep the panel small. It was clear from the outset that establishing and running the panel successfully would be resource intensive, since effective working relationships based on rapport, shared trust and respect would have to be developed. Although we tried not to have any preconceived ideas about how the panel would operate before we discussed it with members, our original intention was for the panel to meet as a group. However, when panel members were approached for suitable dates, times and venues to meet for the first time, two panel members with dementia expressed a strong preference for meeting on a one-to-one basis since they found group situations difficult. One person with dementia was very deaf and found any group situation particularly stressful. They both explicitly said that they would be happy to contribute on a one-to-one initially, although they were willing to review this at another time. Both carers, however, were happy to participate in a group discussion, although one carer who is physically frail expressed concern over possible transport arrangements. This presented a dilemma to the researchers. From past experience, groups have the advantage of facilitating discussion and debate and providing a forum to share ideas and experience. However, if we had been inflexible in our approach, and gone ahead with a group format, we would have effectively marginalised and excluded people with dementia, the very people we were keen to include.

There is some evidence that older people with dementia do not contribute easily in a mixed group (Kitzinger and Barbour 1999). A group situation with people with dementia, carers and 'professionals' might militate against their equal involvement. We considered establishing separate panels for people with dementia and carers. However, the people with dementia had expressly said that they did not wish to meet as a group and separate panels would have considerable implications on limited resources. There was not any strong theoretical reason why the panel had to meet together. We therefore decided to meet with panel members individually, respecting the preferences and prior commitments of the individuals with dementia. Panel members identified preferred times and days for visits and we try to stick to set routines.

The researcher is in weekly contact, either meeting up, or via telephone and postal links. Any documentation is usually sent through the post for the panel to read at their convenience and discuss with each other and then followed up with a personal visit from the researcher. Table 5.2 shows a log of the contact with a panel member and activities over a period of twelve weeks. This is intended to illustrate the type, purpose and intensity of contact between panel members and the researcher.

Table 5.2 Log of activities over twelve weeks

Date	Type of contact	Purpose
22/2/00	Phone call	Social contact
23/2/00	Phone call	Arranged visit
1/3/00	Visit a.m. (1 hour)	Discussion on qualitative interviews, topic guide; reviewed consent
2/3/00	Letters and information posted	Information about project to date; draft topic guide
7/3/00	Visit a.m. (1.5 hours)	Discussion on topic guide
8/3/00	Phone call	Social contact
14/3/00	Phone call	Arranged visit
16/3/00	Visit a.m. (2 hours)	Discussion of topic guide
28/3/00	Visit a.m. (1.5 hours)	Discussion of communication techniques for interviews
29/3/00	Visit a.m. (1 hour)	Discussion of communication techniques for interviews
6/4/00	Phone call from panel member	Cancellation; next visit rearranged
11/4/00	Visit a.m. (30 minutes)	Revision of topic guide
12/4/00	Phone call from panel member	Clarification about topic guide; visit arranged
18/4/00	Phone call	Checking time for visit
19/4/00	Visit a.m. (1 hour)	Finalising of topic guide
25/4/00	Letter	Detailing project progress to date
26/4/00	Phone call from panel member	Clarification of project progress to date
2/5/00	Visit a.m. (15 minutes)	Delivery of project documents
9/5/00	Phone call	Social contact; arranged visit
10/5/00	Visit a.m. (15 minutes)	Review of consent

What does the panel do?

The purpose of the panel and the role of panel members are dynamic and change as the project progresses. The panel helps to decide the important priorities relevant to quality of life for the project team to tackle. It has a key function in helping to analyse, explore and explain the themes emerging from the qualitative interviews (Murphy *et al.* 1998) and to put these themes and issues in a broader context. The data generated from the qualitative interviews is fed back to the user panel, and they help focus on how best to phrase any further questions and discuss overlap and context of these domains. The themes generated from this discussion are then fed back into the next qualitative interview.

This process is, of course, inherent to qualitative research and is an exercise that the researcher would have undertaken in the absence of a user panel. However, the presence of the panel facilitates discussion and helps to ensure the interviews are grounded in the lived experience and views of people with dementia and not skewed towards the interests of the researcher or what is emphasised in the literature.

There have been cases where the interpretation or emphasis of individual panel members differs from that of the researchers and other panel members. In these cases, the alternative views are directly fed into later qualitative interviews. The following dialogue illustrates the type of debate generated by the user panel discussions:

Panel member (carer):

What people need is more money. Talking about choice and so on is all very well, but the bottom line is that we need more money.

Researcher: Okay. So say you had more money? What would that do? … How would that affect this person's life? … What difference is that going to make?

Panel member (carer):

Well they could choose, couldn't they? Little things like being able to get a taxi instead of the bus, would make a massive difference to us, especially when you've been used to getting chauffeured all your life. I think we need to ask about it like that…

Researcher: Do you mean when you had a car?

Panel member (carer):

Yes. It would make a massive difference to us, what we could do, where we could go, how long we stayed for and that, you know things like that matter to us, you know, that's what makes a difference and I think you should be asking about that you know in the study.

Researcher: And is that just about money do you think?

Panel member (carer):

I think that's what it ultimately comes down to yes. If we didn't have Alzheimer's we wouldn't have to think like this, but it forces you into a corner, you know. I think what this person is saying is that if they had more cash they would have a better quality of life. Period.

Researcher: Okay, that's an important factor, but it's not the whole story, is it?

Panel member (carer):

Well, no, okay, maybe not, but you know when you come to talk about what makes a difference to us, to people like us, to me and Mike [pseudonym for panel member with dementia] when we're trying to get on the best we can with life and not bother anyone and not make a fuss, it does matter, it does.

Researcher: I'm not saying it doesn't matter.

Panel member (carer):

What do you think, Mike?

Panel member (with dementia):

(pauses) Well, if you have more money it does help yes. …it does, doesn't it? I thought that as well when you were talking. Ask, you know, other…people what they think about it. It's important, I do know that. See what they say. Yes, put that down.

Panel discussions are tape-recorded, supplemented by written notes. Panel members were also given a diary and asked to record any thoughts, ideas or incidents that they thought might be useful to the research. The consultations are relaxed and informal, but are more structured than a 'little chat', which implies superficial or trivial conversation. Panel members draw on their experience and knowledge. The panel relies on verbal communication although the researcher does not generally dominate the dialogue. The discussions with people with dementia and carers are different. One person with dementia talked unprompted for much of the time and at great length and on some occasions tired easily. There sometimes seems a fine line between people acting as research subjects and as user panel members. However, an advantage of one-to-one discussions is that the power balance is more shared and people with dementia, carers and researchers have a more equal voice in the discussion.

How have panel members found the process?

The ability of panel members to engage in the discussions varied. On some occasions people with dementia and their carers might be 'having a bad day':

Panel member (carer):

> When you came yesterday we'd had a bit of a difficult morning…there were tears and all sorts…and by then we were both just exhausted I think. We didn't know where to put ourselves, never mind think anything through.

However, panel members were generally quick to ring and cancel or rearrange a visit from the researcher, should they not feel like taking part. This illustrates that they felt comfortable with the relationship and were able to exercise choice and control over their involvement in the process.

The fact that two married couples were on the panel was felt to be a benefit for the individuals involved as they could provide support to one another, share ideas and a mutual sense of involvement. However, the person who lived alone found the process more difficult:

Panel member (with dementia):

> I want to help, of course. But it's difficult remembering everything. It's nice to see you though.

This individual needed a lot of reassurance but contributed to the panel in a positive way:

Panel member (with dementia):

> I think it's tricky getting people to talk about this [quality of life]. I think, myself, speaking as someone who has got Alzheimer's...I don't know what it means....if you ask about one thing at a time, I think I can...manage that a bit better, you know.

The panel members who have dementia feel that their involvement has been particularly therapeutic, in that it was the first time that any interest had been shown in their views. Participating in research has been cited as a positive outcome in itself (Bahro, Silber and Sunderland 1995).

Panel member (with dementia):

> When I was first told I had Alzheimer's, I felt useless... I've got more confidence now and even though there is not a cure for what I have I feel I'm...contributing in some way.

It has also been suggested that people taking part in research feel they are contributing to the future and the process of involvement also helps to meet activity, attention and social needs (Gwyther 1997).

Panel member (with dementia):

> It might, you know, help others, further down the line.

Panel member (with dementia):

> It's helping me think, and I need to...that helps me

Panel member (carer):

> Oh, we're happy to help in any way we can. We enjoy it. And if we can help others in the future, well that's great isn't it.

Actually being involved in the panel caused all participants a great deal of anxiety and stress at the beginning, although they were keen to mask this.

Panel member (with dementia):

> When [carer] says you're coming, I look forward to it. I

> have to think hard, and I find that quite tiring, but I like helping.

Panel member (with dementia):

> When you first started coming, I used to worry and that you know [researcher: and now?]. I didn't let on… Oh, I enjoy it now. I feel I've got something to say and can help and that.

Panel member (carer):

> It's given us a chance to think things through, not just look at us internally, but think about lots of other things…lots of other issues…and I hope that helps you.

Benefits of the user panel to the research

The panel has provided a forum and opportunity to share ideas and experience. It has ensured that the research is focused on topics that are relevant and appropriate to the target group. But the panel also helps in explaining the importance of these topics in context and the relationships between them. It has had a major impact in terms of the direction of the research by facilitating a person-centred approach to data collection and helping researchers to find meaningful and appropriate ways to ask questions of people with dementia (Gwyther 1997).

A major benefit of the panel is that it keeps the researcher in touch with the realities of living with dementia. It is easy for researchers to be 'cut off' from such realities and once an initial period of data collection is over, the themes and domains identified can appear rather abstract and detached. However, through regular contact with panel members, the research team has continued to ground the research in the day-to-day experiences of a person with dementia and their carers, and how this changes over time. This has been enormously beneficial to both the researchers and the research.

An additional benefit stems from the panel being formed so early in the project. A key reason for establishing a user panel was to assist in reviewing and evaluating the relevance and appropriateness of existing outcome measures for quality of life. While the panel found it easy to understand the broad aims of the project, and the need for outcome evaluation in principle, they found the technical aspects of outcome measurement particularly difficult to comprehend. An advantage of being involved so early is that they had time and space to understand the topic and so when asked to take part in more challenging exercises reviewing the actual measures, they felt able to take part:

Panel member (with dementia):

> I didn't know what you wanted you know. I didn't know what it was we were doing here. I knew about everyday things and that, like, but these? [outcome measures] right up until June [six months in] then the penny clicked... Oh aye, I'm champion now like, so long as you keep us on all right you know and tell me each time.

This relatively long period of uncertainty and lack of clarity about what is expected has been reported in previous studies (Tozer and Thornton 1995). At the beginning, we tried to be explicit about the panel's role in the project. In contrast to more emancipatory and participatory research frameworks, the aims, objectives and research design were already decided when the user panel was established. In this respect researchers controlled the research. However, the panel developed a supportive role to the research.

Although perceived to be beneficial, the process of the user panel is challenging. It is resource intensive, especially in terms of panel members' and researchers' time. Keeping panel members abreast of developments in the project is also a challenge and it is important to focus on what panel members can do and wish to do. The voices of people with advanced dementia are not represented on the user panel, although they are included in the qualitative research project. However, based on our very positive experience to date, the panel is to be expanded to include people with more advanced dementia for the next stage of the project and four individuals have been approached to take part. We intend to undertake an evaluation of the user panel. This will include reviewing panel members' expectations and the opportunities for the panel to criticise the research and influence future directions.

Summary

People with dementia and their carers can be meaningfully involved as participants on advisory or user panels.

Researchers need to be flexible and responsive in the methods and techniques selected to involve people with dementia.

People with dementia can make a significant contribution to the research.

Active partnerships between people with dementia and researchers through consultation and collaboration are being used to empower people with dementia and their carers to become more involved in research, to monitor and evaluate the effects of their involvement, and to develop models for identifying and prioritising relevant and appropriate outcomes. The user panel described in this paper is exploring exactly how and when members would like to be involved; methods for communicating with people with dementia; identifying and prioritising topics for investigation; and is involved in designing and evaluating the content and form of available outcome measures. The user panel has successfully involved older people and their carers in the research process. It is guiding the development of research tools, and ensures that the voice of people with dementia is directly incorporated in the research project.

Useful contact addresses

Quality Research in Dementia Advisory Network:

The Alzheimers Society Quality Research in Dementia Programme
c/o The Dementia Group
The National Hospital for Neurology and Neurosurgery
London
WC1N 3BG

http://www.qrd.ion.ucl.ac.uk/

Consumers in NHS Research:

Consumers in NHS Reasearch Support Unit
Help for Health Trust
Highcroft
Romsey Road
Winchester
Hampshire
SO22 5DH

www.hfht.org/ConsumersinNHSResearch

Acknowledgements
Dr Lynne Corner is funded by an Alzheimer's Society Research Fellowship.

Thanks to the project user panel; Richard Harvey, Lesley McKinnen, Rachel Litherland at the Alzheimer's Society and QRD Advisory Network, Claire Bamford, Monica Smith, Maureen Craig and John Bond.

References
Alzheimer's Society (1999) http://www.alzheimers.org.uk/

Bahro, M., Silber, E. and Sunderland, T. (1995) 'How do patients with Alzheimer's disease cope with their illness? A clinical experience report.' *Journal of the American Geriatrics Society 43*, 41–46.

Barnes, M. and Bennett, G. (1998) 'Frail bodies, courageous voices: Older people influencing community care.' *Health and Social Care in the Community 6*, 2, 102–111.

Barnes, M. and Bennett-Emslie, G. (1997) 'If they would listen...' *An Evaluation of the Fife User Panels.* Edinburgh: Age Concern Scotland.

Barnes, M. and Wistow, G. (1992) 'Understanding user involvement.' M. Barnes and G. Wistow (eds) *Researching user involvement.* Leeds: Nuffield Institute for Health Studies

Bastion, H. (1994) *The Power of Sharing Knowledge: Consumer Participation in the Cochrane Collaboration.* The Cochrane Collaboration Consumer Network, UK Cochrane Centre.

Beresford, P. and Croft, S. (1993) *Citizen involvement: A Practical Guide for Change.* London: Macmillan Press Ltd.

Carr-Hill, R. and Dixon, P. (1998) *Constructing a Database of Examples of Consumer Involvement in Research.* Centre for Health Economics, University of York.

Gwyther, L. P. (1997) 'The perspective of the person with Alzheimer Disease: Which outcomes matter in early to middle stages of dementia?' *Alzheimer Disease and Associated Disorders 11*, 6, 18–24.

Hanley, B., Bradburn, J., Gorin, S., Barnes, M., Evans, C., Goodare, H., Kelson, M., Kent, A., Oliver, S., and Wallcraft, J. (2000) *Involving Consumers in Research and Development in* the NHS: Briefing Notes for Researchers. Consumers in NHS Research Support Unit, Winchester.

Kitzinger, J. and Barbour, R. S. (1999) 'Introduction: the challenge and promise of focus groups.' In R. S. Barbour and J. Kitzinger, (eds) Developing focus group research. Politics, theory and practice, pp.1–20. London: Sage.

Murphy, E., Dingwall, R., Greatbatch, D., Parker, S. and Watson, P. (1998) 'Qualitative research methods in health technology assessment: A review of the literature.' Health Technology Assessment 2, 16.

Standing Advisory Group on Consumer Involvement (1998) Research: What's in it for Consumers? 1st Report of the Standing Advisory Group on Consumer Involvement in the NHS R and D Programme to the Central Research and Development Committee 1996/97. London: NHS Executive.

Tozer, R. and Thornton, P. (1995) A meeting of minds: Older people as research advisors. York: Social Policy Research Unit, York.

PART TWO

The Views of People with Dementia

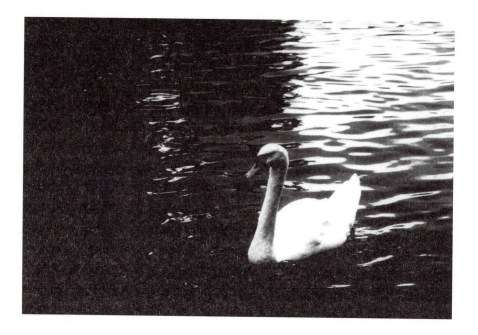

Should people with Alzheimer's disease take part in research?

Elaine Robinson

I think that it would probably be best if I started off by explaining who I am, a little bit about my background, and also how I came to be diagnosed with Alzheimer's disease. My name is Elaine, and I am 45 years old. I have been happily married to Dave for about 28 years, and we have two children – Paul aged 23, and Gail aged 25. I used to work as a staff nurse in a surgical ward in the Edinburgh City Hospital until a severe spinal injury necessitated two operations for slipped discs in October 1995, which were unfortunately both unsuccessful. This left me permanently disabled and I rely heavily on an electric wheelchair when out of doors, although I can get around the house with the aid of a walking frame or elbow crutches.

I was first diagnosed with Alzheimer's disease just before Christmas in 1999. This first came about due to the keen observations of my psychiatric nurse who noticed that I was having trouble recognising coins, and remembering dates and birthdays, during one of her frequent routine visits. After she reported her suspicions back to the psychiatrist caring for me, he came to the house and I underwent a mini-mental test. Later he confirmed to Dave that I had Alzheimer's disease, and had probably had it since I was 42. Dave and I had both noticed that I was forgetting things, but we always put it down to the strong painkillers and the anti-depressants I was taking as a result of my back problem. Now we had something else much worse to cope with. How on earth were we going to do that?

I decided that I was not going to lie down to the disease, or give up. I used to be a dedicated nurse and gave every ounce of my energy and enthusiasm towards helping others. There were still things I could do – turn the tables so to speak, and fight back! I decided that, as I was the youngest person in Scotland with the disease at that time, I would do what ever I could to help raise awareness of early onset dementia. Since being introduced to Alzheimer Scotland I have taken part in many talks and seminars in the UK and I strongly feel that fighting back is by no means futile – I can still do something positive and I'll keep going as long as I am able. This crusade of mine has given me something important to grapple with – maintain my sense of purpose and simply get me up out of my bed when I would otherwise just lie there and get all depressed. Not only that, it also means that Dave and the rest of the family will benefit as they see me feeling stronger, more determined, and a little happier too.

A researcher from the University of Stirling who wanted to interview someone who had just been diagnosed with the disease contacted Alzheimer Scotland. She wanted to find out how they felt during and after receiving their diagnosis, and whether or not they felt they should have been told at all. Alzheimer Scotland then contacted me and asked me if I would be willing to take part in the research – this was right up my street, and of course I jumped at it.

The interview took place in my own home, and Dave was present. I had no idea what to expect but the researcher's warm and friendly manner put me quickly at ease. I find it uncomfortable at times meeting strangers, even when I'm at my best, or taking part in anything mildly stressful, but I must say I found the whole thing very enjoyable. It was, in a way, good for me to talk about how I received my diagnosis to someone other that Dave. When I talk to him about my illness I'm looking for his love, understanding and support, but it's just between us. Talking to the researcher was giving me a chance to say exactly what it was like for me, not just the good points but the bad ones too. Knowing that the results might help a wide range of people understand more about what it's like to receive a diagnosis of this horrible disease made me feel like I was doing something really worthwhile.

There had been something, which had happened just after my diagnosis, that caused a great deal of torment to us both and I wanted it noted by the researcher – something I should never have been exposed to. After receiving the diagnosis from my psychiatrist I just couldn't accept that it was happening to me. This was an 'old' person's disease, wasn't it? I felt so well, I was too young, surely I must have been misdiagnosed? We both lost a great deal of sleep over the news as you might expect. It took a long time for me to begin to come to terms with it, but gradually I started at least to take the first few positive steps on my journey with the disease.

Things were soon to be thrown into turmoil however when my GP disagreed with the psychiatrist's diagnosis when we went to see him. He said that my poor memory was due to the fact that my brain was now relatively inactive and had become sluggish. I left the doctor's surgery on a high – this was just what I wanted to hear. I couldn't understand, however, why Dave didn't share my feelings of elation. The whole thing was deeply troubling him and I later found out that he and my daughter had gone back later in the week to see the doctor to question him further. It must have been hell for them. Apparently the doctor was very dismissive about the entire thing and said that he had no doubt at all what was causing the problem. He swung arrogantly in his chair and threw his hands behind his head and said that the cause of my memory problem was due to alcohol abuse. After all, the liver function tests proved it. He told Dave that I would have by now become very skilled at hiding bottles of booze and was probably buying it at the shops when he was at work. He wasn't with me every minute of the day so I had every opportunity to get hold of alcohol. Yes, according to the GP, I was now an alcoholic!

So there we were – caught in the middle of a difference of opinion between two doctors. Dave was livid and wrote to the practice manager, and had to attend a meeting with him to air his grievance. We eventually got the whole thing sorted out and the GP was made to apologise to us in writing – but it meant that I had to go through the whole painful process again of accepting that I have Alzheimer's disease. It really was a dreadful experience and caused a considerable amount of misery, not just to me but our whole family. We have since moved to another GP, at a different practice, and things are much better now.

If we sufferers are going to be included in any kind of research and given everything we have to help fight this dreadful disease, it would be reassuring to know that we have at least a well informed and approachable GP behind us as part of a multidisciplinary team.

I really think that people like myself should be encouraged to take part in any research and made to feel that their contribution, no matter how small, would be greatly valued. After all, who else would know what it's like to have the disease? No doctor, no matter how eminent, could ever truly appreciate how we perceive the horrors, which lie in wait at times in our often fuzzy and confused world, unless he or she suffers from it too. We often experience the disease in different ways, to a greater or lesser degree, and at different rates of progression. What a wealth of hidden personal experience the skilful researcher can tap into. I also think that we should be encouraged to involve ourselves in research as often as possible, as long as we find it comfortable to do so, during our journey. If I am still able to put my thoughts down on paper or to speak about my feelings and opinions – why shouldn't I be included?

It doesn't follow that as soon as you are diagnosed you immediately become incapable of communicating. Many of us may have many years of good quality life in front of us in which we can still be productive and make a valuable contribution to Alzheimer's research.

What a hugely missed opportunity it would be if people with Alzheimer's were excluded from the very thing that could be used to gain a fuller understanding of their disease. It would be simply denying us the chance to fill in the gaps that no one else can. I realise that a cure for Alzheimer's disease may still be a long way off. I also know that the research I have taken part in so far will not benefit me personally, but taking part in it has lifted my morale, and I'm sure anyone else who has done the same will agree. To know that there are many dedicated people out there, who are willing to take the time and visit us in our own familiar surroundings to listen and record our opinions, makes all the difference.

There are times of course when it is simply impossible for me to take part in anything. Apart from the gradual mental deterioration associated with Alzheimer's I often succumb to sporadic episodes of confusion which may last for just a day, or as much as a week, and to varying degrees of intensity. At times like this the muscles in my face become quite stiff and I find it very difficult to talk and eat. All I want to do is sleep, and I'm afraid when that happens everything just grinds to a halt for me and I rely heavily on Dave to tend to my needs. In a strange way however I do feel quite lucky. That might sound like a weird thing to say but that's how I look at it. I have a young fit husband with great reserves of stamina who has told me often that he will care for me at home for as long as he possibly can. He supports me in everything I do, and I know I can rely on him. Knowing this fills me with great confidence and motivates me.

On my good days I will give all I've got. I will take part in anything and do all I can if I think that somewhere at some time it will help others to beat this awful disease. I realise that it will be totally different for some of the more elderly sufferers. It may be that for many of them there does not seem to be any point in taking part in research. Perhaps they are too advanced in the disease to focus their minds, or suffer other ailments associated with the natural ageing process, which would hinder their efforts. I must say I can't blame them for not taking part.

Then there is the problem of actually recording our thoughts and opinions. It's one thing giving a verbal account of how we experience the disease to a researcher, but it's a totally different thing when we are asked to contribute something in writing such as writing this chapter. It is vitally important that anyone with the disease is given as much time as possible to prepare and produce something of that nature. The last thing we want is to find ourselves becoming agitated as a result of the pressure of trying to meet some impossible deadline. I am fortunate to have my own personal computer, although I now find it extremely difficult to type even the shortest passage and I rely heavily on my husband to do all the typing. At first I tried to record my thoughts using a tape recorder but all I ended up with was a collection of muddled statements which were a nightmare for him to arrange into chronological order. I found that for me, it was easier to make simple notes as they came into my head, which could be seen at a glance, and sorted out later. For those who do not have access to a computer or indeed someone to help collate all the information for them, then things will be much more difficult, or even impossible. So for many, it will not be appropriate to be involved in producing written material.

Feeding back the results and findings of any research to those who took part is crucially important too. It would be very disheartening for us to spend our time taking part in interviews or providing written material only to find that we no longer hear from those conducting the research. I was fortunate to be invited to a seminar at the Quaker meeting house in Edinburgh a few months after I had taken part in the research done by Stirling University.[1] I was asked to speak to those attending about how I received my diagnosis and how I felt afterwards. To say I was nervous doesn't even come close. I was terrified! I'm not used in any way to talking to large numbers of people, and I found it hard to keep my notes from shaking. Once I got started though, I soon found that I no longer needed to refer to my notes. I just told my story as it happened and my apprehension just melted away. I would urge anyone who is asked to speak about his or her Alzheimer's disease to get up, and speak up, and be heard. It's time to fight back not just for ourselves but for those who will no doubt follow us in the future. I found the comments and debate that followed extremely informative, and made contact with several people there who asked me to do other talks for their particular projects – it was all very exciting.

One of the most exciting things I was ever involved in for Alzheimer Scotland was the time Dave and I were interviewed on camera with Lenny Henry. It was for Comic Relief in 2001, and we spent a whole day filming on Arthur's Seat in Edinburgh and another day in and around our home, during the October of the previous year. It was really fantastic being part of something that would go a long way to raising awareness of Early Onset Dementia. Although the filming took two days, the finished piece lasted a mere five minutes. Apparently, when it was shown on air, the telephone lines erupted. It was so wonderful – to see something happening as a direct result of simply speaking up for oneself, and others too. What made it even better was the fact that the BBC had flown Dave and me down to the television studios in London to watch the show. We met many celebrities and got their autographs, and spent the rest of the night with them in the hospitality room.

I hope my contribution to this book has in some way inspired others, who like me have had their lives turned upside down by Alzheimer's disease. It's a devastating thing to have to face but we can do it with dignity, and a voice. It is imperative, though, that we have a GP whom we can trust and rely on, especially when things become more difficult. There's lots of other help and support out there for us too. Alzheimer Scotland is like a huge safety net beneath Dave and me. It's good to know they're there, and all the associated outreach personnel, who are only a phone call away.

I will continue to speak up for myself for as long as I possibly can. I urge you, if like me you have been diagnosed with Alzheimer's disease, to do the same. No one but us knows what it's really like. I would feel terribly annoyed if we were denied the opportunity to take part in any kind of research into a disease which is gradually tearing apart my life, and my husband's too.

Note

1   The study entitled 'The experience of diagnosis from the perspectives of people with a diagnosis of dementia.' (Grantholder Heather Wilkinson.) Funded by the Mental Health Foundation (UK).

Chapter Seven

Did research alter anything?

James McKillop

I was still in the throes of the aftershock of being told I had dementia, the world stopped all of a sudden, when I asked to take part in research.[1] The researcher was asking the question 'Do people have a right to be told they have dementia?' In the past, well-meaning conspiracies sprang into action to 'protect' people from the truth. But could this have had an adverse affect? These cloak-and-dagger activities may have increased the torment of those who knew something was wrong and imagined the worst but kept silent to shield their family. So everyone kept quiet.

Up until then I had never knowingly met another person with the illness and so, never having had the chance to compare case notes, my opinions were unbiased. At least in hospitals you get the instant opportunity to compare lengths of scars and estimates of how much was removed and have the anticipation of telling all and sundry how bad it was, embellishing the story each time naturally.

Rebekah[2] came to my home in the role of the researcher, gently coaxing answers with her thumbscrew set. It was fairly painless although the proceedings did resurrect bitter memories as it had been anything but plain sailing up to then. Being unaware of my condition had led to a very difficult lifestyle and family tensions, and the scars still oozed blood. I was in my own wee world comparable to Dante's Hell, completely bewildered and unable to make sense of anything going on around me.

But enough of that, we all have our own crises to deal with as we journey through life. However, we need the best information so that we can deal effectively with them. I was free to supply or suppress any information whenever I wanted during the interview. Rebekah, a glutton for punishment, was to come again, by then being just about part of the family. Everything was of course confidential on both sides, so I can't reveal Rebekah liked biscuits and cats. She was a little late the first time she came and I thought, 'no wonder, having come all the way from New Zealand'.

I was made aware that a fair number of other people were being asked to participate and the results were to be published. I am as yet unaware of the findings and nuances of the final report, but I suspect my story is typical.[3]

Being told of the diagnosis at the right time, in the right place, by the right person who has thoughtfully allowed plenty of time for explanations and any questions is essential. The diagnosis has to have time to sink in and does affect one's life – for better or for worse. Most people can start to confront a problem once they know and understand exactly what it is. If not told the blunt truth, or if the issue is fudged, you are still in the dark, weaponless, fighting the unknown.

Armed with background knowledge, one is able to assess the battleground. The inner one fighting against the diagnosis (it must be someone else's, it simply can't be mine…) and the worldly one (the world hasn't changed but you have). You now have to come to terms with your illness, learn to adapt to your new limitations and be prepared to meet challenges, for they will surely be there. However, help will be at hand through Alzheimer Scotland – Action on Dementia, and Turning Point Scotland to name but a couple.

In my case there were three paths I could have followed. First the status quo. I could have kept blundering around my shrunken world deeply depressed, as I had been decisively excommunicated from a misunderstanding society. Next I could have simply given up and been watered, fed and lived in limbo until my dying day.

Finally I could stand up to the condition. How dare it think it can control me; I'm still in charge; parts of my brain are dead and/or damaged but I can resourcefully use the remaining working parts to circumvent many of the problems caused by the illness. And I believe that by taxing your brain daily you can delay its progression. It's a losing battle in the longer term, but I'll go down fighting all the way.

About this time I was fortunate in meeting Brenda (a worker at Turning Point) who, using her own time and influences, steered me towards a fresh start in life. I currently receive person-centred help from Turning Point Scotland who put their money where their mouth is, helping people overlooked by society to rejoin society as participants not dependants, as players not spectators. They stand sentinel for the needy.

Rebekah and Heather were co-hosting a conference[4] in Edinburgh to present their initial findings. I was invited along, mainly as I had been involved in the research, but somehow I ended up being scheduled to give a small talk. I was intrigued when I was told that another person with dementia would be there. I had often mused over what they looked like. I wondered how they hid their horns? (I used to grind mine, but after a slip with a Black and Decker and losing memories of 1965, I opted for a pumice stone, which now keeps me looking sleek.)

The wait was worth it, I was very pleasantly surprised to meet Elaine and listen to her experiences, many of which struck a chord. She looked like a glamour model and, as it turned out, she is a model – a role model – telling others how it is and how she copes, uplifting and encouraging others to emulate her. I never was a public speaker though I had muttered the odd word at meetings like PTAs. Suddenly I was up there speaking to a group of discerning people and operating an OHP. What on earth possessed Rebekah and Heather to allow me platform time? Where had the confidence come from to permit me to give a talk? They certainly went out on a limb, putting their heads on the chopping block if it had gone pear-shaped, and both must be highly commended for their foresight and risk-taking stance.

After being a recluse for some years, how did I manage to talk to an audience? Did dementia block out fears of my making an ass of myself or had my new determination to get on top of my illness forged a new me? I just don't know. Wonders will never cease. I must have struck a chord somewhere. The scouts were out at the meeting and both Elaine and I were subsequently invited to speak at an Alzheimer Scotland – Action on Dementia conference later that year. I also made contacts who were later to invite me to their support groups, when I was looking for opinions on a help card I was producing (for people with dementia when they go solo),[5] but that's another story.

It emerged during the research that not everyone was told of his or her diagnosis initially. For some it was a little later, eventually or never. No doubt some weren't told for very good medical reasons but there seemed to be no logical reason for other non-disclosures. Some of the medical profession would not bite the bullet. Was it fear of exacerbating matters or was it lack of understanding? Were they concerned that their patients' lives would be taken over by the 'services' and their spirits quashed? Quien Sabe?

Remember that people with dementia are often shunted behind the scenes and segregated from society. Placed in groups where they are well looked after, tea, biscuits and TLC; male things like dominoes for men and female things like knitting for women. I don't disparage this; it can be heaven for some, discomforting for others. Dementia, while less common in people in their 40s, can nevertheless start then, but it is a problem to provide services where young and old with differing needs are lumped together. But the winds of change are on their way. The powers that be are finally wakening up to the fact that there is a better way and some are taking the first tentative steps to remedy the injustices suffered by many over the years.

OK so you've been told, so what now? You need time to let things sink in and then decide what to do with the rest of your quality life. As explained above, in the past people with dementia were hidden away from public gaze and left to vegetate. But thankfully that is less the case now. It is now recognised that although the prognosis is downhill and irreversible, the decline can be delayed especially where the brain is stretched, put to regular use, and individuals can learn to find a way round many problems (the Gospel according to James!). There is medication that may help some people with Alzheimer's and hopefully there may be medication some day for other types of dementia.

It was also clear from the research that not everyone had equal access to information about where qualified help could be obtained. Having been fortunate in accessing help from Alzheimer Scotland – Action on

Dementia very quickly and appreciating it, I decided to try and ensure that there was material for others to clutch at in their time of need. So I go round doctors' surgeries and hospitals in my local area, leaving posters and help line cards. I also leave them anywhere else I can, for example, in some churches, community halls/centres and public notice boards. Nowhere is sacred! To me it is senseless telling someone they have dementia and then leaving them guessing what comes next. Materials can pave the way towards greater understanding and sources of help. People with dementia can prove (by their deeds etc.) that there is some form of quality life, and are an inspiration.

Did research alter anything? Remember that when I met Rebekah, it was a fait accompli as I had finally been told of my diagnosis, so was research too late for me? I think not! My experiences (and those of others) will surely shape the future and others will benefit. I also met kindred spirits, gained confidence to face the public and speak out (how can I ever thank Rebekah and Heather?) and you – the reader – have been given the chance to reflect. It is the rare person who has not been, or will not be, touched by dementia through family, friends, acquaintances and work-mates. You are better prepared now. Many people want to help but are unclear how. Hopefully some will now be motivated into action to do 'something'. There is a lot to be done and people's individual talents could culminate in awesome pressure groups.

Should research stop there, having achieved its end? Most definitely not. Being told of a diagnosis in the nicest possible manner is a start. However, the public's views and perceptions are still in the dark ages. Only a few days ago, someone in the medical profession helpfully and politely asked if someone 'demented' like me could…

Attitudes encountered by James	
The 'does he take sugar' do-gooders	
The baby talkers	(Yes I can understand their words but not their attitude)
The whisperers	(Who think normal speech levels might start me off)
The knowledgeable	(Who tell others what I think and how I feel)
The concerned	(Who ask after my health as if I were on a danger list)
The gloom merchants	(Just wait till he…)
The cannots	(You can't do that now or ever, after I just did)
The incredibles	(You manage to go out all by yourself)
The unbelievers	(But you have dementia!)
The monosyllabics	(Who fail to recognise I know longer words)
The wellwishers	(Hope you get better soon)

I have also encountered all the attitudes illustrated in the box above. Can I respectfully ask people to treat us as normal and only make allowances for particular problems. I am constantly telling people that having dementia does not automatically mean you are 'demented' and I have written elsewhere on this vexing problem, hoping it will provoke discussion. I sincerely hope research on this is to follow!

Notes

1   The study entitled 'The experience of diagnosis from the perspectives of people with a diagnosis of dementia.' (Grantholder Heather Wilkinson.) Funded by the Mental Health Foundation (UK).

2   Rebekah was one of the researchers on the project and was originally from New Zealand.

3   The Final Report 'Tell me the Truth' is available from The Mental Health Foundation and will be distributed to everyone who took part in the research. www.mentalhealth.org.

4   This was a one-day event held on 12 October 2000 to feedback the findings from the research to participants and local service providers.

5   The helpcard and guidance on how to use it are now available through Alzheimers' Scotland-Action on Dementia, 0131 2431453.

PART THREE

Methods and Motivations

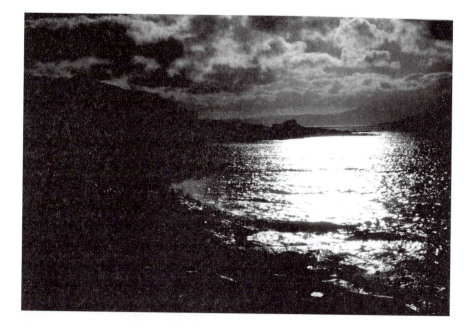

Working with staff to include people with dementia in research

Kate Allan

Introduction

The material in this chapter is based mainly on my experience of undertaking the work which resulted in the book *Communication and consultation: Exploring ways for staff to involve people with dementia in developing services* (Allan 2001). This study followed on from work started in Stirling by Malcolm Goldsmith, which culminated in his book *Hearing the Voice of People with Dementia: Opportunities and Obstacles* (1996). A description of the work I undertook is provided below. As well as arising from this experience, what I have said here is also based on my background as a clinical psychologist working with older adults. In this role I worked with staff in various kinds of service settings. Although this had a clinical rather than research emphasis, it nevertheless taught me a great deal about the possibilities and constraints within which one must operate.

The project

The aim of the study I carried out between May 1998 and October 2000 was to explore the process of staff undertaking service user consultation with people with dementia. At this time old attitudes about dementia destroying the person's ability to communicate were giving way to more positive and realistic views, and the centrality of communication to good care practice was gaining recognition (Goldsmith 1996). By the time the study got underway service planners and providers generally were becoming aware of the need to develop ways of involving people with dementia in the design and delivery of services, and to find out more about their experiences of using them. Legislation and policy was quite clear on this point (for example, Department of Health 1990, 1994; Filkin 1999). Earlier research studies (Barnett 2000; Dabbs 1999; Lam and Beech 1994; Phair 1990; Proctor, 1998; Sperlinger and McAuslane 1994; Sutton and Fincham 1994) had demonstrated that people with dementia did have opinions and preferences regarding their care and could, with the right kind of support, express these to others. However, all of this work had been undertaken by personnel external to the service in question, and this separateness was emphasised as a way of encouraging people to say what they really thought. Clearly, however, if service user consultation is to become an integral part of the relationship between the user and the provider, then this work has to be done by those who actually deliver the care. And so this provided the direction for the most recent phase of the work.

The study was a small-scale, exploratory attempt to look at how staff could encourage those in their care to express their views, opinions and needs. The focus was firmly on the process (how we could help people to express opinions) rather than the outcome (what people said about services). The part of the study discussed here involved nine services where 40 members of staff worked with 25 people with dementia. The services that contributed to the work were identified as settings that had already demonstrated a commitment to innovative and progressive work, and many of the staff who participated were especially interested in communication and were willing to accept the challenge of being involved. The contributing services and staff therefore were not a typical group, but in order for the study to make some progress in the time available, it was felt that a 'fertile ground' approach was justifiable.

The participating services included day, residential and long-term nursing care settings. No home-based services were included, mainly for pragmatic reasons since organising research within these settings presented more challenges than we were able to meet within the scope of a relatively small and short project. However, we recognise this as an important gap since so many people with dementia already receive services in their own homes, and this is a growing area. The staff who took part were a mixed group. The largest number were unqualified social care and nursing assistant staff. Some psychiatric and general nurses took part and there was one occupational therapist. The people with dementia who participated were also a very mixed group. Efforts were made to include people with quite severe levels of disability overall and significant communication problems. Some were largely non-verbal, and some engaged in behaviour that was considered challenging.

The study utilised a new approach to consent, which attempted to keep the person with dementia more at the centre of the process. It is not possible for reasons of space to go into detail about this aspect of the work here, but the interested reader will find a fuller description in Allan (2001).

In some of the sites the active fieldwork phase (when staff tried out various approaches to communication and consultation) lasted for almost ten months. In other services, which got started much later, this period was as short as six weeks. In all of the sites the aim was to generate and try out approaches to communication and consultation that were tailored to individuals or small groups of individuals. Aside from some very general initial ideas about what could be done, which had arisen from Goldsmith's work (for example, providing opportunities for one-to-one conversations, group activities and discussions, studying non-verbal communication), the canvas was fairly blank. It was in discussions with staff, once we had identified individual people with dementia who were going to participate in the project, that more specific approaches were shaped up.

This was done by talking to staff about the participants themselves, their personality and background, their strengths, needs and preferences as regards communication, and by thinking about the kind of relationships they already had with the practitioners who were going to undertake work with them. The overall aim was to build on the positive aspects of these. Ideas for starting points were developed, and then staff tried out the various approaches. Following on from their efforts there were further discussions with myself about what had happened. As a consequence of these discussions approaches were sometimes repeated or developed, sometimes they needed to be modified or new directions altogether found. In this way, the initiatives undertaken by each member of staff, or set of staff if more than one were working with an individual or group, were developmental and highly differentiated.

Work with each participant or group of participants followed its own path, and the progress of initiatives was inextricably linked with their context. This context encompassed factors pertaining specifically to the individual participant (for example their health and well-being, their willingness to undertake work for the project at any one time); factors pertaining to the service setting (such as the deployment of staff, shift systems, routines and activities etc.); influences on staff (including their health and well-being, patterns of working, absences etc.); and the needs of other service users.

Clearly the combinations of these contextual factors created a very complex picture into which work for the project fitted. This meant that the initiatives that were pursued took a very variable course. In some cases work with an individual participant or group of participants was conducted in a reasonably smooth and continuous way. But in most instances there were ups and downs in terms of how consistently work could be undertaken. Some of the participants experienced periods of illness (either related to or independent of their dementia) or were otherwise unavailable for project work. Some of the staff had periods of absence from work during the fieldwork phase, and these limited the extent to which initiatives could be developed. Sometimes the absence of staff in other parts of the service meant that those who were participating in the project had to change their role to cover for their colleague, and this constrained what could be achieved. Some services went through periods of organisational change, or increases in demand for what they were offering meant that there was no spare capacity with which to undertake work for the project.

Although, at one level, such influences could be seen as obstacles to the progress of the research, an alternative way of viewing them was simply to accept that all of these factors combined to create the reality of the world of services. Most of the events and influences that arose during work for the project were not especially unusual – similar things were going on all of the time. This meant that these were the conditions in which staff normally had to operate. Understanding, accepting and working within these constraints and opportunities was actually a core objective of the project. If, after all, the whole enterprise was going to yield outcomes that were useful to ordinary service settings, they had to derive from conditions that were comparable to real situations.

I have organised the material in this chapter by discussing issues as they arose in the course of working with staff, with more general points being discussed towards the end.

Values inherent in the work

Before embarking on collaboration with staff it seemed important to clarify in my own mind the kinds of values that would underpin my work with them, and also to share these with the staff. These ideas were first discussed at introductory workshops (described below) with staff, but were also reinforced throughout the collaboration.

The first was that we were approaching this work without anyone, especially myself, having the role of 'expert'. I wanted to make it clear that my assumption was that everyone had important knowledge, skills and insights to contribute, and that much of the progress we were hoping for would come about through my learning from the staff about what they were already doing, rather than it all being about my teaching them to do new or different things.

Another important point was that as far as possible the experience of contributing to the project should be enjoyable and valuable for the staff; that as well as sharing their own knowledge and skills, they, and therefore their service users, should derive benefit as well.

Developing relationships with staff

The first point to make here is that it takes time, and almost always longer than expected, to reach the point at which the kind of relationships that will support collaborative working have developed. This must be allowed for in the time schedule. Trying to get going before proper partnerships are in place is likely to lead to problems later.

Getting off on the right foot is also very important. In the case of my own work, following on from agreements with managers in the various services that we would go ahead (and again time was necessary to reach this point), arrangements were made to meet the staff who would potentially do the actual work. This was done by organising a (two–three hour) workshop session in each setting. The purpose of this was to introduce myself as the researcher, and the context and aims of the project, and to begin to develop relationships. Both the managers and I were keen to involve as many staff from each setting in the workshop as possible, even though the expectation was that a much smaller number would go on to participate directly in the work. The rationale for this was to promote general understanding of the nature and purpose of the study and to get as many staff as possible interested in what we were doing. It was felt that this would provide the best conditions for some to take part more specifically.

The workshop sessions were kept as relaxed and informal as possible. Aside from introducing myself and providing people with information about what I was doing, I was keen to encourage staff to share their own ideas and experiences. I did this first of all by asking them to say what the term 'dementia' meant to them, and how working with people with dementia made them feel. This was intended to project the message that I was interested in them as people, and in the meaning of their work to them. We then went on to talk about the subject of communication generally, followed by an exercise where staff were asked to think of a recent encounter with a person with dementia which had gone particularly well. The intentions of this exercise are described further below. Although in-depth discussion of the practicalities of the project was kept to a minimum on this occasion, one important component of the introductory workshops was to reassure staff about the scope of what they might be getting involved in. With ample justification they were concerned about extra workload and how compatible it would be with their existing duties.

Discussions about this formed part of what was to become an on-going dialogue about the whole enterprise of research, and how it related to practice. It is important to recognise that until recently practitioners and researchers have occupied worlds that hardly overlap at all. It is to be hoped that this is now changing, but each, with its own kinds of specialist knowledge and skills, rules and language, can present as rather intimidating and confusing to the other. Since this book is concerned to some extent with research in service settings – meaning that we as researchers are going out into the world of practice – there is a particular need for us to offer information in a form that is digestible and timely for practitioners, and to provide opportunities for them to express and explore any concerns about what they may be taking on.

In the case of my own work, it was not too difficult to reassure staff about what was expected of them. But it was also necessary to be honest about the fact that the research work would be focused on their practice, and might therefore pose challenges to their attitudes and actions. How exactly this is tackled by others will depend on the nature and aims of the research and the methodology being planned. Whether or not participation by staff is voluntary will also be an influential factor. In the early stages of a collaboration there will be a need for sensitivity to different sorts of reactions from staff. Some may embrace the prospect enthusiastically, whilst other will be more cautious. Reluctance, scepticism or even hostility towards the idea may mask apprehension, anxiety, or feelings of being threatened. It is vital to provide opportunities for people to express and discuss such reactions. Some people may have had negative experiences of research in the past, and require reassurance that whatever led to the sense of disappointment will not be repeated.

Helping staff to become aware of what they already know and do

The success of the work I did depended completely on the willingness of staff to undertake initiatives, report back and then develop the work. Further, one of the fundamental assumptions of the whole enterprise was that these practitioners already knew and practised a lot of what we were trying to pin down. It was therefore vital to support staff in reflecting on and talking about their existing resources, and then finding creative ways to build on that.

However, I have found that staff who are experienced and skilled in what they do are often very modest in their estimation of their own contribution, even when things are going well. Some of this may have been attributable to a reluctance to seem over-confident, and because discussions took place, at least initially, in a group setting. However, I am sure that many of the practitioners did find it genuinely difficult to recognise and value their own resources and skills properly. This may be due in part to the low status of care work generally, or it may be that the use of skills and knowledge to promote good communication become so overlearned and automatic in the course of using them from day to day that it is difficult to see them as being distinctive and special.

Whatever the reason for this tendency, it was important for the research that we did try to identify what it was that was already going on, both so that we could plan more opportunities for staff to do what seemed to work best, and also so that the self-esteem and confidence of staff could be heightened. As mentioned above, one of the ways I did this was to ask practitioners (at the introductory workshop) to think of a recent encounter with a service user that they felt had gone especially well. I asked them to describe it in detail, and encouraged them to try to identify what it was they had done to bring about such a positive outcome. Almost all of the staff found this difficult to do. They expressed the view that they had not done anything special, but rather that what had occurred in the interaction had been by chance or due to factors external to themselves. It was necessary to examine these incidents in some detail, and to break the intervention of the practitioner down into small steps in order for all the knowledge, sensitivity and judgement used to become apparent. Once we had done this, however, it seemed to be the start of a process of bringing these skills into more conscious awareness, which then allowed further development to take place.

Getting to know services

It seems a very obvious thing to say, but in order to pursue a realistic collaboration it is vital to learn as much as possible about the settings in which a piece of research will take place. This can be done in two main ways – talking to managers and staff and spending time in the setting with staff and service users. The process of talking to staff and managers was discussed above in some detail, so here I will concentrate on the matter of spending time in service settings.

For much of the kind of research this book is concerned with, the methodology may include the allocation of time in the care setting, perhaps doing observation work or working directly with people with dementia. Obviously such time will be an integral, and maybe substantial, part of what is being done. In addition to this, however, it is important to devote some time simply to being in the environment where the research is taking place, and interacting with the people who are there in an unstructured way. Although such a commitment may be given a particular name, such as induction or familiarisation time, aside from this it seems helpful to approach it without a specific plan or agenda. With the agreement of staff and service users, the objective is simply to be there and to take part in whatever is going on at the time.

When there was a great deal else to do, it could seem somewhat wasteful to allocate time to this process, but in my case I believe it paid real dividends. On one level it allowed me to absorb some of the atmosphere of the places, their rhythms and routines, and the way that their character could vary over time. I believe that not having any particular focus for my attention helped me simply to be open to what was going on, and probably resulted in my becoming aware of important factors that affected what we were setting out to do or the ways we went about it.

Getting to know the people with dementia and inviting them to get to know me was also of central importance. Although we now appreciate that everyone who develops dementia is an individual, and that the interaction of the condition with their pre-existing uniqueness results in further differentiation, there is no substitute for actually just being there and encountering people for who they are. At the same time you have the opportunity to let people get to know you. Being around without having any particular task or focus means that I simply had to present myself as I was. At first this seemed threatening, and did arouse certain feelings of anxiety. Without the protective shield of, say, a clipboard and rating form, how would I know what to do, what to say, how to respond? Such feelings are understandable and survivable. Drawing on values and habits such as sensitivity and tact, and respect for people's feelings and privacy helped and taught me more of what I needed to know. Sometimes the only way to gain confidence is to get out there and do it.

There is another potential benefit in getting to know service users. It may have been that once staff realised that I was interested in the people they were working with, and had some understanding of who they were as individuals, they perhaps felt more confident and comfortable about sharing details of their experiences in working with them. They were able to see that I was not afraid of people with dementia, and to observe my strengths and needs in terms of the ways in which I communicated with individuals. This did feel exposing, but I felt that if I was prepared to be honest about my starting points and open to learning from them, then the resulting conversations with staff about care work, about dementia as a condition and about the persons affected by it were more likely to reach new levels of profundity. Through doing this I believe that I was in a better position to make sense of what they said and did, generally and as part of the research, and to help them to gain a deeper understanding of my concerns and objectives.

Another important reason for spending time in service environments was to demonstrate to staff that I was willing to share the space in which they work, that I was not somehow above or remote from it. Practitioners' previous experiences of researchers may have been of people who floated in and out of the setting, who seemed interested only in a very narrow slice of what went on, and who simply took away information whilst giving little or nothing back. For research to be truly collaborative and mutually beneficial there needs to be much more give and take, and devoting time and energy to participating even in a small way to the life of a service is one way of giving something back.

Involving staff in the design and carrying out of work

The work I did was to a large degree reliant on the knowledge and skills of staff for coming up with ideas for approaches to communication and con-sultation, and obviously since they were doing the direct work, I was dependent upon them actually to carry it out. It was therefore vital to involve them as much as possible in the process. This took place within the many conversations I had with staff over the period of the project. I made a point of asking them for their opinions as to how we should go about doing things, and what support they needed from me, and I took their advice as to the feasibility of certain approaches. I sought their opinions on the usefulness of resources such as pictures, objects and other stimuli for conversation and interaction, and tools such as recording forms. I asked them about how appropriate, accurate and relevant the written feedback given to them was, and whether they needed anything else from me in order to continue and develop the work.

Apart from the fact that this was the only practical way to pursue the collaboration, another effect of this was probably to increase the practitioners' sense of ownership and involvement in what was happening, and looking back on it, what I seemed to be doing here was, by involving and consulting them as much as possible, providing a model for the involvement and consultation of people with dementia.

Control vs. collaboration

As researchers we start out with a vision for what we want to know, and how we will go about finding it out. Constructing proposals for funding, submissions to ethics committees and so on demands a great deal of forethought and planning and preparatory work. Throughout all of this, ideas about how things will unfold are taking shape in our minds. It is impossible to anticipate everything, however, and adjustments will always have to be made, fallback plans brought into action, and sometimes even major rethinks. All of these conditions apply even when you as the researcher have the maximum possible degree of control over what is happening. When the success of the enterprise depends on collaboration with others, it is a very different story.

It is important to accept at the outset that in making the involvement of staff an integral part of the work, a large number of new factors, many of which will be largely unknown before the collaboration has begun, will be introduced. Although the sorts of things which will figure in this may be anticipated (for example one may expect that the attitudes and emotions of practitioners will influence how things develop), until the enterprise is actually underway it is unlikely to be clear what these are and what their consequences will be. This means that timescales and plans have to be constructed with the inherent complexity and unpredictability of service settings and their personnel in mind.

What staff need from a researcher

In my own work with staff it was very important to give as much time as possible to talking about what we were trying to achieve together. The kind of talk that took place during the project had various forms and served various sorts of purposes. An important point is that not all of the discussion centred specifically on project-related concerns. The fact that the study was rather loosely defined, and therefore did not have clear edges, contributed to the need for talk that was more wide-ranging, since it would have been difficult to predict from the outset what was going to be relevant and what was not. However, this was only one of the arguments in favour of setting up these sorts of opportunities for talk with staff. The main aim of the project was to explore the process of undertaking service user consultation with people with dementia. For this to happen in the most meaningful way, it was important to have set discussion of the more specific details of the work in the context of staff, reflecting on the nature of their work in general, their own personal sense of meaning in doing it, and the feelings and reactions it generated in them.

Where talk was more focused on care practice and project work, I found that bringing staff together in small groups was most likely to generate discussion that was significant and instructive both for myself, as the researcher, and for them. It was often apparent that during such occasions practitioners shared and gained the kinds of insights that seemed to open up new ways of understanding the words and actions of service users, and their own role in helping people to express themselves. This often came about through members of staff telling their colleagues about incidents, conversations and exchanges involving service users, which they had either participated in or observed. This kind of storytelling prompted others to remember other occasions that were similar or different, and the practitioners discussed the ways in which they had made sense of these incidents, and how the incidents had influenced their perceptions of people and the way they communicated with them.

I am convinced that it was these sorts of conversations, which arose and unfolded very naturally with only a little prompting and encouragement, that really helped to open up understanding, stimulate ideas and move things on in terms of the research. But I also became convinced that staff need far more opportunity to do this kind of thing in the course of their usual practice.

Fitting in with their routines

In work such as this, which occurred over a period of time and took a developmental form, ways of keeping in touch were of central importance. The sites that took part in the project were scattered quite widely over the UK, so frequent visits were not possible. Talking to staff on the telephone and providing written information and feedback were the main modes of contact.

It is not possible to go into a great deal of detail here, but having phone contact with the staff proved to be a very interesting aspect of the methodology. Many of the services operated on a shift system, so it was necessary to get to know how these worked and keep up to date with rotas in order to increase the chances of being able to reach the right member of staff at the right time. I developed an elaborate timetable of phoning during the fieldwork phase. Evenings and nights were the best times to talk on the phone. Daytime calls were always more rushed and busy. The main thing was to fit in with when the member of staff was able to come to the phone, and although a shift may last nine or ten hours, the best times for a phonecall may have been only one 30-minute slot within that. Sometimes, even then, plans for a conversation did not work out if something unusual had occurred in the setting or it was an unexpectedly busy time. Sometimes I did not manage to call at the appointed time, or could not get through because the phone was engaged. When calls were missed, for whatever reason, this often posed challenges to the continuity of our efforts since many of the staff worked part-time, and may not have been back in the setting for another four or five days. Maintaining adequate phone contact was one of the biggest challenges of the whole thing.

Responding quickly

Because what we were doing was so intimately tied up with the ups and downs of the well-being and health of the person with dementia, the availability and energy of the practitioner and the complexities of services themselves, it was in the nature of the work that I, as the researcher, had to be as flexible and responsive as possible when opportunities for trying something out presented themselves. There were many times when there was a great rush to send out a picture or specially designed form or written information about something so that the member of staff could try an approach the next day, before going on leave or having a spell working in another part of the service.

Providing feedback

In order for the staff to gain the most from their experience of taking part, it seemed important to provide prompt and specific feedback on their efforts. This was a vital part of the exercise, and was often the stepping stone to what came next. All of the feedback that was provided was personalised and tailored as much as possible to the needs of each member of staff, and the work they were doing. Remaining alert to the practitioner's need for feedback, even if it was not as formal as that described above, seemed very important. As we shall discuss below, it often takes a great deal of courage for staff to take the step of trying out something new.

Receiving prompt feedback and reassurance that their efforts were appreciated and useful was a crucial way of acknowledging the staff's commitment and helping them remain interested and motivated in taking the next step. This point is particularly important in the context of studies that involve a large number of staff. Although from the busy researcher's point of view it is all too easy inadvertently to leave someone out in terms of feedback, it is most unfortunate if someone is left feeling that he/she is the only one who has not been recognised for his/her efforts.

In other sorts of studies it may not be possible to work with staff in this way for reasons that are integral to the design of the research. In any case, though, it will be important as far as possible to clarify exactly what staff can expect in the way of contact and feedback as they go along, and what will be forthcoming at the end. It goes without saying that such agreements must be honoured, even though from the researcher's point of view this can be difficult, since by the end of the period of active collaboration there is a sweep of tasks to be completed, which can be rather incompatible with going back to settings and giving feedback. This is discussed further below.

Boosting self-esteem and confidence

It seemed to me that there was particular need on the part of practitioners for reassurance and discussion when it came to taking the step of trying something new. It is easy to underestimate how much courage it takes to launch out in a novel way. At such a time all sorts of different feelings may be brought into sharp focus – lack of confidence about skills and knowledge generally, feelings of confusion or uncertainty about the study itself, concerns about possible negative effects of the new approach on service users, fears about being shown to have failed if something does not 'work', worries about what will be revealed if it does (this was a particular concern in my case, since the study involved asking service users about their opinions of the care they received). There are many possibilities, and time must be allowed for discussion of these sorts of concerns throughout the process. This may be done on a group basis, but some practitioners may be more comfortable sharing their concerns more privately. Some people may have difficulty identifying and talking about such issues at all, but their misgivings may express themselves in their actions, such as by non-cooperation, questioning or challenging the point of the exercise etc. Again, as researchers we must be alert to this sort of possibility, and be open to ways of dealing with it.

Using our own experiences to enhance understanding of the person with dementia

One of my main interests in work with people with dementia is in their subjective experiences – what sorts of thoughts and feelings people have when they are struggling to find a word or carry out a task, how they feel when they realise that others are treating them differently, and how having dementia affects their whole view of themselves and who they essentially are.

Since the study I carried out was about finding ways of learning about the experiences that people with dementia had of the services they used, it seemed useful to try to use our own experiences of carrying out this work to try to gain a deeper understanding of what was happening to the people we were working with. Talking to staff about the possible similarities between their own experiences and those of service users, and people with dementia generally, was one way of doing this. And since the experience of taking part in a research project was new to most of them, this seemed a logical place to start. The fact that the study was loosely defined in terms of both its aims and methods meant that the potential for feelings of confusion among the staff who contributed was strong.

When these feelings arose, I tried to be aware of them and to talk to staff about what was happening. Once we had established that it was entirely understandable that they should be feeling unclear about what it was they were supposed to be doing, the links between the qualities of their own experiences and those of service users could be explored further. This approach seemed to work well both as a way of reassuring people, and in opening up possibilities for discussions that went fairly deep into the nature of dementia as a condition and its meaning for those who used the service. Although talk of this kind took practitioners' feelings about the project as a starting point, it is likely that there are also many feelings generated in the course of routine care work that could be examined for their similarities to the experience of people with dementia. This way of thinking about our own experiences could be developed further as an important way of learning more about the subjectivity of those with the condition.

Finishing up

This is the phase of a research process that is most likely to be poorly planned and executed. It follows on from what may have been a long and very busy period of work. Once the active phase of collaboration is over, there may well be a rush to produce outcomes for publication or presentation. One's mind is liable to be focused on a whole range of other priorities. Attending to the details of the closing process, and making sure all the loose ends are tied will probably be a considerable challenge, but I believe, for a variety of reasons, that it is extremely important to conclude the period of collaboration in a way which does justice to what has been done already, and maximises the possibilities for mutual learning.

Feedback exercise

A key part of the closing process in the case of my own research was providing staff with the opportunity to give feedback on their experience of taking part in the research. This was done by designing a questionnaire that both asked specific questions and provided space for staff to write about the aspects of the collaboration that had been most relevant or striking to them. On account of the relatively small number of staff participants, and the individualised nature of the work they had done, it was clear that there would be little point in aiming for feedback to be anonymous. It therefore seemed rational to make a virtue of personalising the exercise as much as possible. This was also in keeping with the other stages of the work.

In the event, practitioners were provided with a carefully designed booklet-style questionnaire which had their own name on it, and included a personalised letter insert which reminded them of the various approaches they had attempted with the service user. A self-addressed envelope was included, and each practitioner was sent a postcard acknowledging the return of their questionnaire. The response rate from those who had had a reasonable degree of involvement in the project was very high (81%), but a decision was taken to invite those staff members who had not, for various reasons, undertaken much work for the project to provide feedback as well. This was justified on the grounds of general inclusiveness, and because of the possibility that practitioners who had not contributed substantively could nevertheless offer valuable insights into the nature of the enterprise, and perhaps the reasons for their minimal involvement. Most of these individuals simply did not return the questionnaire, but their inclusion was amply rewarded by the frankness of one member of staff. In the questionnaire she described her sense of disappointment and frustration when the collaboration in her setting proceeded in such a way as to make any meaningful involvement on her part difficult if not impossible. She apologised for being unable to express more positive thoughts and feelings, but in fact she made a very important contribution to the project. Although it was painful for me to read what she had written (all the more so for the fact that hers just happened to be the first questionnaire returned!), her perspective enabled me to gain insight into the less 'well-lit' areas of the project, and to see how my own ways of understanding what was happening and my own actions had affected how things had unfolded. If I had known at the start what she was going to write in the questionnaire it would definitely have changed the way I went about things through the fieldwork phase.

Since the subject of the work was the experience of staff exploring new approaches to communication and consultation, inviting feedback was a particularly important exercise. A great deal of pertinent information was gained, both about the quality of their experiences, and the effects that participating in the research had had on their attitudes and practices. I also learned more about the context of the work, including the characteristics of service users and service settings that had had an impact on what had been attempted and achieved. Even if the focus of the work had not been so squarely on the experiences of staff, however, such an exercise would have been a crucial part of a collaboration. It could take a variety of forms, and be conducted on an on-going basis rather than waiting until the end of the enterprise.

Written outcomes

Following on from the feedback exercise, and alongside work on other written outcomes of the study, I produced a report for each of the services that had taken part. This document was specific to each site. In each case it was approximately 10,000 words long, and detailed the background of the study, the ways in which the collaboration had begun and developed, and described what work had been undertaken by the staff. It also provided brief discussions of the issues that were raised by the work. I went to considerable lengths to make it readable and visually attractive. It was written so that it could be shown to anyone who was interested (this meant that certain details were excluded and some descriptions kept vague to protect confidentiality). These reports served two main functions: they were a way of bringing together information about the study that could be used both by staff and personnel external to the organisation and they were a tangible piece of evidence of the contribution of the service to the study.

A key part of the process of producing these reports was again consultation with staff. Each person who had taken part was invited to look at a draft of the report and comment on it. Many obviously gave it careful attention, and made astute observation about its content and tone. Even though conducting such consultation hugely increased the amount of work and time it took to produce these reports, I do believe it was worth it. Again it underlined the fact that the perspectives and contributions of the staff were valued, and resulted in a document which the services were proud to show to others as evidence of their involvement.

The final written communication with the staff was a personal and individual letter thanking them for their support of the work.

Conclusions

This chapter has described just one way of going about working with staff in a research project involving people with dementia. Some of its points are more specific to an exercise such as the one I carried out, some of them will be applicable to other sorts of studies.

There are no doubt many other important issues that have not yet been encountered and explored, but I hope this account conveys some of my own sense of excitement about the possibilities that are within reach if we are prepared to find good and useful ways of working together with practitioners. One of the staff who took part in the study said:

It's been a very positive project, which has shown us how much we already do unconsciously but has reminded us to always be aware of the different ways there are to communicate and made us more aware of each individual's choices and right to choose.

Surely it can only be by entering more fully into the practitioner's world – their experiences, thoughts and feelings – and learning from them that we can hope to achieve the kind of understanding and skills we need in order properly to address the concerns and experiences of those with dementia.

Having to make things up as one goes along, not being entirely clear about what is going on presently, not knowing what is going to happen next, and needing to be on the alert for clues and directions forward were all integral to the experience of carrying out this work. Perhaps this is what it feels like, at least at times, to have dementia, and perhaps this is the position in which practitioners find themselves in the effort to provide care. If so, these parallels and shared experiences must be rich in learning potential.

Acknowledgements

I am grateful to the Joseph Rowntree Foundation who funded the work. My thanks also go to the people with dementia who participated in the study and their relatives who supported it; all the staff in the services and the many others who advised and encouraged.

References

Allan, K. (2001) *Communication and consultation: Exploring ways for staff to involve people with dementia in developing services.* Bristol: The Policy Press.

Barnett, E. (2000) *Involving People with Dementia in Designing and Delivering Care: 'I need to be me!'.* London: Jessica Kingsley Publishers.

Dabbs, C. (1999) '*Please knock and come in for some tea': The views of people with dementia and improving their quality of life.* Preston Community Health Council. Available from Preston CHC, 128–130 Miller House, 9 Lancaster Road, Preston, PR1 2RY.

Department of Health (1990) *NHS and Community Care Act.* London: HMSO.

Department of Health (1994) *Working in Partnership.* London: HMSO.

Filkin, G. (1999) *Starting to Modernise: Achieving Best Value.* London: New Local Government Network.

Goldsmith, M. (1996) *Hearing the Voice of People with Dementia: Opportunities and Obstacles.* London: Jessica Kingsley Publishers.

Lam, J. and Beech, L. (1994) *'I'm sorry to go home' The Weekend Break Project: Consultation with Users and Their Carers.* Monograph from Department of Psychology, St Helier NHS Trust, Sutton Hospital, Cotswold Road, Sutton, Surrey, SM2 5NF.

Phair, L. (1990) *What the People Think: Homefield Place from the Client's Point of View.* Monograph available from Eastbourne and County Healthcare, Seaford Day Hospital, Sutton Road, Seaford, East Sussex.

Proctor, G. (1998) 'There's always a difference: They're higher up' *Journal of Dementia Care, 6,* 16–17.

Sperlinger, L. and McAuslane, D. (1994) *'I don't want you to think I'm ungrateful...but it doesn't satisfy what I want.'* Monograph available from the Department of Psychology, St Helier NHS Trust, Sutton Hospital, Cotswold Road, Sutton, Surrey, SM2 5NF.

Sutton, L. and Fincham, F. (1994) 'Client's Perspectives: Experiences of respite care.' *Psychologists' Special Interest Group in Elderly People Newsletter* 49, 12–15.

Chapter Nine

Successes and challenges in using focus groups with older people with dementia

Claire Bamford and Errollyn Bruce

Therapeutic group work with people with dementia is well established (Cheston 1996; Feil 1993; Gibson 1993; Yale 1991) and has demonstrated the ability of people with dementia to work together in groups. In contrast, the use of focus groups to explore the views and experiences of people with dementia has received little attention. Focus groups are an increasingly popular method in social research and have been used to explore a diverse range of topics in a variety of contexts (Barbour and Kitzinger 1999; Morgan 1993; Vaughn, Schumm and Sinagub 1996). It has been argued that focus groups are particularly appropriate for research with people with limited power and influence (Morgan and Krueger 1993), suggesting that they might be a useful way of involving people with dementia in research. The defining characteristic of focus groups is the use of group process and interaction between participants to generate data (Kitzinger and Farquhar 1999). By prompting an exchange of views and opportunities to hear and react to the views and experiences of other participants, focus groups can provide insight into both how and why people think as they do (Morgan 1997).

The aim of this chapter is to reflect on the use of focus groups in researching the perspectives of people with dementia. We begin by looking at the practical tasks of identifying potential participants, obtaining consent, and organising and running the groups. The method is then evaluated by considering the extent to which a focus on the research topic was achieved and group interaction between participants was generated. We also describe the ways in which focus groups with people with dementia differ from focus groups with other participants. The chapter concludes by summarising the strengths and limitations of focus groups as a way of involving people with dementia in research. Since the emphasis of the chapter is methodological, the substantive findings are not discussed here but are described elsewhere (Bamford and Bruce 2000).

Background

A series of focus groups with older people with dementia was conducted as part of a programme of research into the outcomes of social care (Qureshi *et al.* 1998). Desired outcomes of social care were identified through consultations with a range of stakeholders, including older service users, carers, practitioners and managers. Focus groups were organised according to the characteristics of service users and the type of work of staff in order to maximise peer support and encourage frank discussion. Separate groups were convened for older people receiving minimal and intensive levels of home care, with dementia, with functional mental illness, and from minority ethnic groups, and a telephone group was arranged for people who did not leave their homes. Each focus group met several times to allow people to consider the issues, discuss and possibly change their opinions. This deliberative approach (Stewart 1996) was adopted as the term and concept of outcomes were unfamiliar to most stakeholders. For people with dementia, meeting on more than one occasion was also important because of their difficulties in forming cumulative value judgements which sum up all of their experiences (Sperlinger and McAuslane 1993).

In addition to offering a deliberative approach, several potential advantages of focus groups over individual interviews were identified (Table 9.1).

Table 9.1 Potential advantages of focus groups

Increased control over level of participation since there is less pressure to contribute than in individual interviews (Farquhar and Das 1999).

Participants may feel supported and empowered in a group with others who share similar experiences (Morgan and Krueger 1993).

Increased access to memories outside the current context, since sharing experiences might trigger recall of similar events or feelings (Merton, Fiske and Kendall 1956).

Enhanced quality and quantity of interaction in a group context (Bleathman and Morton 1992).

While some benefits are relevant to all research participants, others are specific to people with dementia. In particular, previous studies have shown how people with dementia who rarely communicated during daily routines made articulate contributions to a validation therapy group (Bleathman and Morton 1992).

Practical issues in convening and running focus groups

The ways in which focus groups are set up and planned have a significant impact on the types of people who participate and the data obtained. Our approach to identifying older people with dementia and obtaining consent, and the practical aspects of organising the focus groups are there-fore described. Attention is drawn to the ambiguities and issues that can arise when inviting people with dementia to participate in research.

Identifying potential participants

People with dementia were identified through a specialist resource centre for older people with mental health problems which provides long-stay accommodation, day care, respite care, an outreach team and support for carers. Staff were briefed on the project and asked to identify service users who would be able to participate in group discussions and would be attending for day or respite care during data collection. Staff excluded people with severe cognitive impairments, communication difficulties, people who disliked being sedentary and those who might prove disruptive in a group setting. While staff control over participation was offset to some extent by encouraging other interested service users to join the discussions, only two other people with dementia chose to take part.

Fifteen older people with dementia participated in the study, two of whom attended all five group discussions. The number of service users attending formal discussions ranged from four to nine. All but one participant were female, the majority were in their 80s and eight lived alone. In terms of service use, all but one used day care, five had regular respite care and seven used the home care service.

Carers of potential participants were informed that their relative would be invited to participate and were themselves asked if they would be willing to be interviewed. These interviews provided background information about the person with dementia and carers' views on the desired outcomes of social care for themselves and the person they supported (Bamford and Bruce 2000). These interviews were conducted by a researcher who was not involved in the focus groups and the interview data were not used in the group discussions.

Inviting participation and seeking consent

There is increasing recognition that obtaining informed consent is a complex and difficult process in any qualitative research (Kayser-Jones and Koenig 1994; Mason 1996). Additional ethical issues arise in research involving people with dementia (Bartlett and Martin 2000). Our aim in seeking consent was to ensure that people with dementia had a genuine choice over participation, based on some understanding of the purpose of the study and how the information they provided would be used. We were guided by the consent procedure used with other older people in the outcomes programme. We therefore chose not to seek written consent, particularly since we were concerned that it might create unwarranted anxiety, for example, where people could remember signing an 'official' form, but were unable to remember why. Instead, we relied on verbal and behavioural consent, and stressed that participants were free to withdraw at any point during the discussions. We approached potential participants individually to describe the study and invite them to take part.

The usual practice of seeking consent only at the outset of research has been criticised since consent is not an event but a process (Kayser-Jones and Koenig 1994; Mason 1996). We took the view that attending the initial discussion did not constitute consent to the series of meetings. We therefore invited participants individually to attend subsequent meetings, reiterating that they did not have to attend and could leave whenever they wanted. Continuing consent was sometimes needed during meetings, as illustrated by the following exchange with one participant who had been asleep:

Participant 1:   What am I doing here?

Facilitator: We're all having a discussion.

Participant 1:   I've been listening to all this you see and I thought, 'Well, what am I doing here?'

Facilitator: You've been joining in as well [name].

We used the fourth focus group to feedback our preliminary analyses. We hoped that by illustrating how information from the discussions had been used, participants would be better able to indicate whether they were willing for the information to be used.

Ambiguities and problems with consent

There were ambiguities with the consent procedure, particularly regarding the status of material collected outside the group discussions. On one occasion a service user who had participated in several discussions and seemed to enjoy them, was reluctant to attend. The impression of the facilitator who first invited her was that she seemed uncharacteristically withdrawn and subdued. A second facilitator (a community psychiatric nurse) therefore approached the person with dementia to explore her feelings and reasons for not wanting to participate. After a short discussion, it became clear that she thought she had been admitted to long-term care and abandoned by her carer. The facilitator reassured her that she would be going home after a period of respite care. Following this disclosure and reassurance, the service user decided to attend the focus group.

This example highlights the need for background information about participants and raises important ethical considerations. For whose benefit did we follow up the person with dementia's refusal to attend? Was it for her benefit, because we were concerned about how she was feeling, or for our benefit, because we wanted her to attend the group? What is the status of the information she disclosed to the facilitator? Can this legitimately be included as data, or was it a private conversation separate from the research?

In our view, we did not exert undue pressure on the participant to attend. She had previously chosen not to attend one meeting and we thought she could not easily be persuaded to attend. Our subjective impression was also that she felt better after talking to the facilitator and contributing to the focus group. While the status of the discussion with the facilitator was unclear, the information provided was significant in two ways. First, it confirmed the difficulty that people with dementia had in making cumulative value judgements when their experience varied over time. Second, it provided evidence that within the group we were mainly accessing idealised 'public' accounts (Cornwell 1984). Regardless of whether we explicitly used the information, it influenced our thinking and understanding of users' experiences, by illustrating how idealised accounts presented in the discussions could differ from participants' experiences on different occasions and in different contexts. With hindsight, the facilitator should have asked the participant for permission to share what she had said with the other facilitators and to use it as part of the research.

Exercising choice over participation

Over the series of discussions, a number of participants either decided not to attend or left on-going discussions, confirming that they felt able to choose whether to participate. The ability of participants to withstand pressure to attend was considerable. One participant, for example, consistently declined to attend one discussion even though she was inadvertently approached by all three facilitators and invited to the group. Participants who chose to leave during a discussion often gave socially acceptable reasons for withdrawal, which may have been genuine or a way of leaving without giving offence, for example, going to the toilet or for a cigarette. In contrast, one participant clearly indicated that she had had enough:

Participant 2: I'm going to leave you now.

Facilitator: Well, I think we're going to wind up now, we're just about finished.

Participant 2: Well, we've beaten you to it, the meeting's now closed!

Some participants remained in the room but appeared to withdraw mentally from discussions, although it was not always easy to tell whether participants were concentrating or had fallen asleep.

Confidentiality

A final ethical concern relates to the confidentiality of what is said within the groups. The researcher has little control over how other participants treat the information expressed in the discussion (Kitzinger and Barbour 1999; Smith 1995). In groups with people with dementia, there is the particular difficulty that participants may not remember where the comment was made, or that there was an agreement not to disclose information outside the group. This may be an important consideration in using focus groups where the content may be particularly personal or sensitive.

Organising and running the groups

A series of six meetings, each lasting up to one hour, was planned over a four-week period. One session was subsequently replaced with two parallel informal discussions in the day room. Formal group discussions were held after lunch since participants often sat and chatted informally at this time and no competing activities were scheduled. There were three facilitators at most meetings to ensure that there was always someone available to help participants go to the toilet or return to the day room.

We used simplified versions of a topic guide developed for discussion groups with older people (Table 9.2). We also used a case study and photographs of older people receiving assistance with everyday tasks to prompt discussion. We hoped these stimulus materials would enable us to extend the discussion beyond personal experiences (Schoenberg and Ravdal 2000) and would prompt recall of services received outside the resource centre.

Table 9.2 Topic guide and case study

Main themes on the topic guide:

Views on day and respite care.

Types of help received at home.

The experience of being helped.

Help that might be needed in the future.

Letting people know how you feel about help.

Case study

Jack is 80 and lives alone. He's not keeping on top of the cooking and cleaning these days and doesn't see much of other people. When he had a fall recently, he was alone for hours without any help.

What do you think should be done about Jack?

How might Jack feel about getting help?

How could we find out how Jack is getting on?

What if he got worse and kept falling over, what should be done about him then?

Focus and interaction in the groups

Since two defining characteristics of focus groups are that they have a focus and generate interaction within the group, the extent to which these characteristics were achieved within our focus groups with older people with dementia is considered.

Achieving a focus

We used the topic guide flexibly and often allowed participants to dictate the direction of the discussions, occasionally returning to our initial questions to re-focus the group. The discussions were very broad, and participants often focused on issues that appeared to be 'off-topic'. Much of the discussion was concerned with 'idealised' accounts (Cornwell 1984) or telling stories (Banks-Wallace 1998; Cheston and Bender 1999) and the significance of these is discussed towards the end of the chapter.

Photographs were successful in generating discussion about the experience of being helped, particularly where participants received similar assistance. Furthermore, by describing how the person in the photograph might feel about being helped, participants were sometimes able to move away from idealised accounts and acknowledge some negative consequences of receiving assistance:

Facilitator: What do you think about that chap? Do you think he'd be happy having his hair combed like that?

Participant 3:   Well, I'm surprised that he's allowed it, anybody to come and molest his head of hair in such a manner as this. I wouldn't be at all surprised to hear that he's got up rapidly out of his chair and taken the comb and combed his hair his own way and not someone else's method.

By using photographs of people receiving help in their own homes, we were also able to broaden the discussion to home care. This would not otherwise have been possible, since not all participants could remember whether or not they received help at home.

The case study was less successful in generating discussion and using a male character probably contributed to the poor response. The group consisted almost exclusively of women (only one man participated) and the discussion focused mainly on the issue of gender and the different abilities of men and women to manage. While this provided useful information about the self-perception of the women in the group and their resistance to receiving help, a case study involving a woman, with whom they could more closely identify, would probably have been more productive.

There was some evidence that participants understood the focus of the discussions. After the first few discussions, participants sometimes spontaneously talked to us about services before the focus group was convened. Participants also sometimes reminded one another of the purpose of our visits:

Participant 4: I don't know what they're doing, I can't understand them.

Participant 2: Getting to know our business, that's all.

Generating interaction between participants

Participants interacted in a range of ways during the discussions. Sometimes interactions had a practical focus; for example, where participants encouraged or helped one another to contribute to the discussion, such as by relaying questions to a participant who found it difficult to hear the facilitator:

Facilitator: Does she [daughter] let you do as much work as you want to do in the house?

Participant 5: I can't hear.

Facilitator You can't hear?

Participant 4: Does she let you work at [the] house? Do you do a lot of work at [the] house?

Participant 5: Yes, I might tell you I do a lot of washing-up and I don't like it very much.

Other interactions were more typical of the types of interactions described in focus groups in the literature (e.g. Vaughn *et al.* 1996). Listening to one another often prompted recall of similar events or feelings and led to 'snowballing' or the development of particular themes:

Facilitator: When you felt better after your accident, did you feel like keeping on with Meals on Wheels?

Participant 6: Er no, not really.

Participant 7: It passes the time on making something, doesn't it?

Participant 6: Yes it does, yes, yes. And you do a little bit of shopping for it.

Participant 7: It occupies your time.

Participant 6: Yes, and it takes one of your incentives away doesn't it really?

Interaction sometimes generated useful data, for example, when alternative interpretations of events were offered by other participants. Such interactions were not necessarily positive; for example, one participant suggested a negative and destructive interpretation of events:

Participant 8: I lost a lot of money that I had on one side you know for, you know what happened when I needed money, but when I went to look for it, it had gone.

Facilitator: Gone, how did that happen, how did you lose all that money?

Participant 8: I don't know who did that, but I'm not going to say I can blame somebody, because I can't.

Participant 9: Was it your family, because they're nearest to you, aren't they? They know what you possess and that don't they?

Participant 8: Yes, it could have been my own people, I don't know. [...]

Participant 9: Well it must have been your family that took it.

Participant 8: It must have been dear, there was nobody else in.

Participant 9: Because they had a key to [the] door and they could come in when they wanted, so they're to blame.

Participant 8: Yes, they had, they could come in, they, they, that's it you see.

While the facilitators tried to defuse this, and similar situations, by drawing attention to other possible explanations or points of view, we often found that the same issues arose repeatedly during the discussion.

Another problematic aspect of group interaction was the lack of respect participants sometimes showed one another. This was often manifest non-verbally as, for example, when one participant rolled her eyes at the comments made by another. Such non-verbal gestures could be upsetting if observed. This happened on only one occasion and, fortunately, in this instance the non-verbal gesture did not refer to the speaker, but to another service user who could be seen through the window. It was therefore possible to reassure the speaker that the gesture was not related to him. Although the facilitators valued the participation of people with dementia, the negative responses of other participants could undermine the speaker's confidence and feelings of self-worth.

The supportive nature of focus groups has been highlighted by previous researchers (Banks-Wallace 1998; Morgan and Krueger 1993). Despite the interactional problems described above, the willingness and enthusiasm of most participants to attend meetings suggested that they provided a welcome variation from the usual routine. Participants said discussions had been enjoyable and supportive:

Facilitator: Do you enjoy listening to other people's stories?

Participant 10: I think it sometimes does you good to listen to what other people have to put up with.

Participant 7: I think so too.

Participant 10: When you think that you're all alone in the world, you find out you're not.

Distinctive features of focus groups with older people with dementia

In designing and implementing focus groups, accepted principles or procedures are sometimes modified to make this approach more appropriate for specific groups of participants (Stewart and Shamdasani 1998). While some of the difficulties we experienced in using focus groups are common to many studies, others have rarely been reported in the literature or have a particular salience in relation to research with people with dementia. Distinctive features of our focus groups with older people with dementia are therefore considered here (Table 9.3).

Table 9.3 Issues in using focus groups with older people with dementia

Familiarity

Context

Background information on participants

Domination by one or two individuals

Parallel conversations

Idealised accounts

Story telling

Interpreting data

Familiarity

Participating in research is a new activity for most people with dementia and we aimed to make the focus groups distinct from usual activities but at the same time ensure a sense of continuity and familiarity where possible. The specific strategies used to achieve this balance and avoid overwhelming people with dementia and generating anxiety were:

> holding the focus groups in a familiar setting
>
> meeting participants informally beforehand
>
> inviting a member of staff to the initial meetings
>
> using ritual to frame the discussions.

While neutral venues are often recommended for focus groups (Krueger 1993), other researchers have argued that there is no such place and that instead consideration be given to the likely impact of the venue on participation (Bloor *et al.* 2001; Kitzinger and Barbour 1999). We chose to hold the discussions within the resource centre since this was a familiar environment and participants would already be physically assembled. Formal discussions were held in an unfamiliar room, a short walk from the day room. This proved disorienting for participants; they were often unsure where they were and indeed whether they were still at the day centre, as in the following exchange:

Participant 3:   I think it's still on the wall in the passage from the...

Facilitator: Yes, I think we saw it, didn't we?

Participant 3:   ...from the present.

Facilitator: From the dayroom, yes.

Participant 3:   Dayroom, through to, beyond the, the, beyond the, facing the, in the barracks.

Facilitator: I know where you mean though.

Participant 3:   Yes.

Facilitator: That passage all the way through, yes.

Participant 3:   Yes it's, it's a very long arduous passage is that one.

Although participants were already at the resource centre, the process of convening the group was often protracted. On one occasion, for example, a participant came to the room where discussions were held, decided to leave, was brought back by staff and left again before the discussion began.

Basing the discussions within the resource centre also meant that participants generally knew one another, at least by sight, but they were not a cohesive pre-established group. Disadvantages to using participants who already know one another include the potential impact of an established pecking order on participation and the possibility that participants will feel constrained by their on-going social relations with other group members (Bloor *et al* 2001; Greenbaum 1998; Michell 1999; Vaughn *et al*. 1996). There are also advantages to using pre-existing groups (Kitzinger 1994) and we thought the reassurance of being with familiar faces outweighed the potential problems. Three distinct subgroups of participants could be identified. Some were individuals who did not consistently identify with any particular group within the day centre, others belonged to a group of day care users who habitually sat in the 'smokers' corner of the day room, and the remainder belonged to a separate group within the day centre who consistently sat together. As in previous studies (Kitzinger 1994), we found that some participants from the latter group would only attend meetings if other members of this well-established group were also invited.

Since the facilitators did not know any of the participants prior to the group discussions, we arranged to meet potential participants informally over lunch before the first discussion. We also invited a member of staff with a special interest in group work to attend the initial discussions as a familiar face for participants. Although it was not possible to evaluate formally the impact of her presence on the discussions, no significant differences were noted in the content of the discussions according to whether the member of staff was present or not.

Ritual was used to frame the formal group discussions and delineate them from usual routines and activities (David 1991). A similar format was followed each time, we wore similar clothes for each visit, and created a characteristic smell in the meeting room by burning essential oil. The meetings were framed by offering sweets and singing. Staff suggested singing since it was a popular activity with participants. The opening song was usually followed by a period of complete silence during which we formally introduced the group session, reminded participants about the aim of the research, and requested their participation and their permission to tape-record the session. The chairs were arranged in a circle, with the tape-recorder on a small coffee table in the centre.

It is difficult to assess the extent to which our efforts to make the sessions distinctive from normal routines were successful. Our subjective impression is that they helped participants to remember who we were and why we came to the day centre. For our group, singing was particularly pleasurable and proved enormously helpful in easing the transition to a new environment and activity.

The significance of context

The importance of consulting people with dementia in private, to ensure they are able to voice any criticisms or make personal disclosures which they do not want staff to overhear, has been stressed (Sperlinger and McAuslane 1993). Arranging consultations, or focus groups, in a separate room, however, removes physical cues from the environment that may help participants to recall their experiences. One participant, for example, contributed little to a discussion on hairdressing, but when walking past the hairdressing salon with a facilitator said:

Participant 4:   I'm not going in there am I? They're always messing
                 about with your hair.

One potential approach to resolving these tensions between privacy and recall, would be to use photographs or a video of participants themselves receiving services, either within a communal setting or in their own homes.

Participation in a focus group or individual interview may provide a welcome distraction from usual routines and activities, resulting in the expression of predominantly positive views. We therefore explored the impact of context by replacing one scheduled formal discussion with two smaller, informal discussions with established groups in the day room. One of these informal discussions began as a one-to-one interview, and then broadened into a discussion as two other service users joined the conversation. The other was a discussion with a small group of women, most of whom had participated in at least one formal group discussion. Participants were more critical of services in the informal discussions in the day room and we were able to explore views on on-going activities and reasons for not participating. The informal discussions in the day room also facilitated participation of people with dementia who had not attended the formal discussions because, for example, they disliked being sedentary.

Additional benefits of informal discussions with established groups related to group process. Some of the problems experienced in the formal discussions were minimised in the informal discussions involving groups of participants who regularly sat together. For example, we experienced fewer problems with pacing or parallel conversations and participants were more respectful to one another. However, the informal groups were still dominated by particular members, and communication norms may be more strongly exerted in pre-established groups (Kitzinger and Barbour 1999).

Consistent with previous studies, we found it more difficult to control the agenda in the informal groups (Green and Hart 1999). A separate concern relates to the issue of consent; while in the formal and informal groups it was possible for participants to leave, in the informal groups some participants might have stayed despite not wanting to contribute because there was nowhere else for them to go. In this situation, it was therefore particularly important not to put pressure on anyone to participate (Green and Hart 1999).

Background information about participants

Usually within focus groups, the facilitator has little information about the characteristics of participants before the meeting. Since people with dementia could not necessarily recall their living arrangements or services received, access to such information was essential. This enabled us to ask specific questions of people who attended for respite care, used day care several times a week or who lived alone. Such information was helpful in managing group process, for example, by moving the discussion away from dominant participants and providing an invitation for quieter members of the group to contribute.

Background information was also essential to enable the facilitators to respond accurately to questions participants asked during the group discussions. While it was sometimes appropriate to reflect questions back or ask other participants for their views, the questions often merited a direct response (Oakley 1981):

Participant 4:   What day is it today?

Facilitator: It's Tuesday, isn't it?

Participant 4:   Tuesday, oh we go home today, don't we?

Facilitator: You do, go in the bus today.

Participant 7:   I don't know whether I'm going home or not.

Facilitator: I think you're stopping aren't you? For a few more days.

Domination by one or two participants

Domination by one or two vocal participants is often an issue in focus groups (Bloor *et al.* 2001; Greenbaum 1998, 2000; Krueger 1998) but may be particularly problematic in research involving people with dementia. The memory problems experienced by people with dementia mean that discussion tends to focus on topics raised by the facilitator or other participants, since this triggers recall of similar experiences. Other factors that are equally, or more, important may not be recalled or discussed unless prompted by the facilitator or stimulus materials. There may therefore be more potential for a dominant participant to exert a significant effect on the findings in group discussions with people with dementia.

There were undoubtedly dominant individuals in our group discussions. The fluid composition of the groups helped to avoid consistent domination by a single individual. Background information about participants was useful in managing dominant participants; for example, by asking whether others in similar situations shared the same views, or inviting participants from different backgrounds to contribute their experiences. Stimulus materials were also useful in refocusing discussion and involving other participants.

While techniques such as holding up one's hand, making a 'shh' gesture, or ignoring the individual have been suggested as ways of managing dominant participants (Greenbaum 1998, 2000; Krueger 1998), these met with limited success. This may partly reflect established group norms, where one participant routinely dominated conversations and therefore continued to do so within the context of the formal discussions.

Parallel conversations

While the focus groups successfully generated interaction between participants, it was also common for participants to talk simultaneously, resulting in several parallel conversations rather than a group discussion. Although previous studies have suggested that this is particularly likely in large focus groups (Vaughn *et al.* 1996), we experienced problems with parallel conversations independent of group size.

Careful listening to the recordings indicated a number of reasons for parallel conversations. Sometimes participants suddenly thought of something that they wanted to contribute and did so, regardless of whether anyone else was already speaking. It was clear that we were seen as people who were interested in listening and participants almost invariably addressed such comments to one of the facilitators.

The facilitators themselves sometimes instigated parallel conversations due to the difficulties in pacing the discussion. While respondents can take as much time as they need in an individual interview, in a group context it was more difficult to wait for responses (at least for the facilitators). It was not always clear whether silence was because the person did not want to respond, had nothing to say or was still working out what to say. This difficulty in interpreting silence sometimes led a facilitator to invite several people to respond to a question, resulting in a series of parallel conversations as participants formulated their responses.

Strategies for coping with parallel conversations have been used in therapeutic groups, and might be appropriate in group discussions. For example, the speaker may be handed a scarf, and others are asked to wait to speak until the scarf is passed to them. To help recall, participants may communicate the point they want to make to a facilitator, who then 'holds' the comment until it is the person's turn, and then, if necessary, reminds the person of the point he/she wished to make (Heller 1998).

Idealised accounts

Focus group data represent only one of many possible accounts of the lives and experiences of participants. Previous researchers have described the ways in which participants may put on their 'best face' or offer 'idealised' or 'public' accounts in interviews and focus groups (Cornwell 1984). The use of idealised accounts varied according to the topic under discussion, the context, and between individual participants. We did not seek to discover the 'truth' or otherwise of particular accounts, but considered how they might provide insight into participants' values and the stress points in their lives (Jarrett 1993).

While other researchers have described how participants may challenge idealised accounts in focus groups (Jarrett 1993; Kitzinger 1994; Morgan 1993), this rarely occurred in our groups with people with dementia. Idealised accounts were however sometimes contradicted by observation, informal conversations or subsequent contributions by the same participant. As described earlier, one participant's distress at apparently being abandoned contrasted with her previous reasoned justification for respite care:

Participant 7:   If somebody's been looking after you for twelve months or so, I think they're entitled to have a rest.

During a formal discussion, one participant emphasised her independence:

Participant 8:   I keep my damned house clean. I keep everything clean. I do it myself. I don't ask for anybody coming in.

However, in a subsequent informal discussion, she acknowledged the difficulties of managing on her own:

Participant 11: It's a shame what can happen to you as you're getting older... Well, same as coping with your work at home. It's hard work isn't it? Really hard work.

Participant 8:   Oh it is. Then you complain to yourself. You're talking to yourself, I do – 'Come on, you lazy bitch. Get off your backside'.

Participant 11: I tell myself that, more or less.

Participant 8:   I said – 'If I could kick myself up [the] backside, I would do it'.

The emphasis on idealised accounts may have been due to the fluid group membership, resulting in a lack of safety and cohesiveness, the 'outsider' status of the facilitators (as people without dementia), individual and group norms regarding communication, or the way the groups were facilitated.

There were strong conventions regarding communication among some group members, which essentially took the form of 'mustn't grumble'. Participants were rarely observed to request the help of staff even when they needed assistance. This reluctance explicitly to seek help was reflected in idealised accounts, which typically emphasised participants' ability to manage on their own.

While participants openly discussed the help needed because of other physical or sensory impairments, the needs and difficulties arising from their cognitive impairments were rarely acknowledged or discussed. This may reflect the perceived legitimacy of these needs or group conventions against explicitly discussing their cognitive impairment.

Although different facilitation skills or techniques might have been successful in challenging these established patterns of communication, the disruptive effect of dismantling established coping strategies needs to be considered (Cheston and Bender 1999). Since we were not available to deal with the aftermath of encouraging the participants to confront and discuss the realities of their lives, more challenging facilitation techniques might not have been appropriate. While some authors have successfully integrated therapeutic components within focus groups (Cohen and Garrett 1999), we were concerned about managing the transition between these different modes of facilitation.

Story telling

While idealised accounts were concerned with the present, participants also spent considerable time telling stories about the past. Interview studies with people with dementia have described the use of story telling and suggested that the role of the interviewer is to listen and try to understand the story and identify the meanings that lie behind the words (Barnett 2000; Sperlinger and McAuslane 1993). Three functions of story telling have been identified (Cheston and Bender 1999):

> to create an identity for oneself
>
> to create a sense of interdependency
>
> to explore and make sense of current experiences.

Stories fulfilling each of these purposes were identified in the group discussions. One participant often recounted stories about times when she had the upper hand, such as in this interaction with a doctor:

Participant 10: He said 'Well, when did you last mix with anybody?' I said, 'Good God I did, I did nursing for years and I had to mix with all sorts of people' I said 'including doctors

> like you'. He said "You don't think much of me, do
> you?" I said 'Well, you're all right in small doses'.
> [Laughter]

The interpretation of some stories was therefore relatively straightforward. In contrast, it was not always clear whether other stories were communicating something about the current situation (Barnett 2000; Cheston and Bender 1999) and/or fulfilling some other purpose, for example, catharsis or bonding with other participants (Banks-Wallace 1998). These more ambiguous stories were told by a small number of participants, sometimes more than once:

Participant 5:   My mother was a reader. My grandma never went to school but she taught herself to read and my mother used to tell a story that after tea they'd be sitting by the fire and there'd be my grandma with her head in a book, and my mother, and my grandad used to get fed up of trying to have a conversation. So in the end, he used to get so mad he used to go round and knock all the books up, so they'd all lost their places and then he used to say 'Well, I'm off out'.

The participant who told this story had a severe hearing impairment and this story was, perhaps, a way of communicating her experience of trying to participate in a group discussion.

Interpreting data

Although much of the discussions superficially appeared to be tangential to the topic guide, careful consideration of accounts and stories contributed significantly to the analysis. In considering the meaning of the idealised accounts, desired outcomes could often be deduced by the contrast between the idealised accounts and participants' present situation.

In general, we were cautious about interpreting metaphors. One difficulty in interpreting stories was that potential meanings were often only identified later and it was difficult subsequently to check our interpretation with participants. We had hoped to use the feedback session to check our interpretation with participants and resolve any queries. This proved impractical, however, since participants did not always recall comments or stories they had told.

Analysis of the group discussions indicated that the themes identified were similar to those identified in previous interview studies with people with dementia (e.g. Lam and Beech 1994; Sperlinger and McAuslane 1993). Furthermore, the outcomes identified by people with dementia were generally consistent with those identified by other older people (Qureshi *et al.* 1998). We were therefore confident in the quality of the data and our interpretation.

Summary

Our experience of using focus groups confirmed that this approach can be successful with older people with dementia. The extent to which a *focus* was achieved varied, and there was a strong emphasis on idealised accounts and story telling. Careful consideration of the resulting data, however, indicated that much of the discussion was pertinent to the research topic. In particular, contrasts between the accounts and stories presented by participants and their current situation provided insights into the desired outcomes of older people with dementia. While *interaction* between group members was generated, the group sometimes fragmented into a series of parallel or sequential conversations. Nevertheless, many of the benefits of focus groups were realised, for example themes were developed through discussion, and recall of similar experiences or feelings was triggered by listening to other participants talk. Significantly, participants experienced the groups as a supportive way of contributing to research.

Using focus groups with older people with dementia was also challenging. Adapting focus groups to accommodate the specific needs and difficulties that characterise dementia enabled many of the problems to be minimised. In particular, the setting of focus groups and recruitment of participants had a significant influence on the content and process of the group discussions. The use of pre-existing groups reduced problems of group process, although established communication norms probably inhibited discussion of certain topics. Using a series of groups was beneficial since there was less pressure to cover all of the topic guide within a single meeting, participants could express different viewpoints on different occasions, and membership could be adjusted over time to develop a group which worked well together. Stimulus materials proved useful in managing group process and accessing other settings. Finally, feeding back the results to participants enabled us to illustrate how the information was being interpreted, and to validate and thank the people with dementia who participated.

The advantages and limitations of focus groups have been described elsewhere (Morgan and Krueger 1993; Stewart and Shamdasani 1998) and these should be considered in selecting the most appropriate methodology to answer specific research questions. Focus groups are only suitable for researching certain topics with some people with dementia. Where focus groups are appropriate, however, they can provide rich data on the lives and experiences of people with dementia.

Acknowledgements

This work was undertaken by the Social Policy Research Unit which receives support from the Department of Health; the views expressed in this publication are those of the authors and not necessarily those of the Department of Health.

References

Bamford, C. and Bruce, E. (2000) 'Defining the outcomes of community care: The perspectives of older people with dementia and their carers.' *Ageing and Society 20*, 543–570.

Banks-Wallace, J. (1998) 'Emancipatory potential of storytelling in a group.' *Image – The Journal of Nursing Scholarship 30*, 1, 17–21.

Barbour, R. S. and Kitzinger, J. (1999) 'Afterword.' In R. S. Barbour, and J. Kitzinger, (eds) *Developing Focus Group Research: Politics, Theory and Practice*, 200–201. London: Sage.

Barnett, E. (2000) *Including the Person with Dementia in Designing and Delivering Care: 'I Need to be Me!'* London: Jessica Kingsley Publishers.

Bartlett, H. and Martin, W. (2000) *Ethical issues in dementia care research*. BSG Annual Conference Proceedings September. Oxford: Oxford Brookes University.

Bleathman, C. and Morton, I. (1992) 'Validation therapy: Extracts from 20 groups with dementia sufferers.' *Journal of Advanced Nursing 17*, 658–666.

Bloor, M., Frankland, J., Thomas, M. and Robson, K. (2001) *Focus Groups in Social Research*. London: Sage.

Cheston, R. (1996) 'Stories and metaphors: Talking about the past in a psychotherapy group for people with dementia.' *Ageing and Society 16*, 579–602.

Cheston, R. and Bender, M. (1999) *Understanding Dementia.* London: Jessica Kingsley Publishers.

Cohen, M. B. and Garrett, K. J. (1999) 'Breaking the rules: A group work perspective on focus group research.' *British Journal of Social Work 29*, 359–372.

Cornwell, J. (1984) *Hard-earned Lives: Accounts of health and illness from East London.* London: Tavistock.

David, P. (1991) 'Effectiveness of group work with the cognitively impaired older adult.' *American Journal of Alzheimer's Care and Related Disorders & Research* July/August, 10–16.

Farquhar, C. and Das, R. (1999) 'Are focus groups suitable for "sensitive" topics?' In R. S. Barbour and J. Kitzinger (eds) *Developing focus group research. Politics, theory and practice*, pp.47–63. London: Sage.

Feil, N. (1993) *The validation breakthrough: Simple techniques for communicating with people with Alzheimer's-type Dementia.* London: Health Professions Press.

Gibson, F. (1993) 'What can reminiscence contribute to people with dementia?' In J. Bornat (ed) *Reminiscence reviewed: evaluations, achievements, perspectives.* Buckingham: Open University Press.

Green, J. and Hart, L. (1999) 'The impact of context on data.' In R. S. Barbour and J. Kitzinger (eds) *Developing focus group research: Politics, theory and practice*, pp.21–35. London: Sage.

Greenbaum, T. L. (1998) *The Handbook of Focus Group Research.* Second edition. London: Sage.

Greenbaum, T. L. (2000) *Moderating focus groups: A practical guide for group facilitators.* California: Sage.

Heller, L. (1998) 'Working with the Wednesday Group.' Presentation to the Psychotherapy and Dementia Special Interest Group, September, University of Bradford.

Jarrett, R. L. (1993) 'Focus group interviewing with low-income minority populations: a research experience.' In D. L. Morgan (ed) *Successful focus groups: advancing the state of the art*, pp.184–201. London: Sage.

Kayser-Jones, J. and Koenig, B. (1994) 'Ethical issues.' In J. Gubrium and A. Sankar (eds) *Qualitative Methods in Aging Research*, pp.15–32. London: Sage Publications.

Kitzinger, J. (1994) 'The methodology of focus groups: The importance of interaction between research participants.' *Sociology of Health and Illness 16*, 1, 103–121.

Kitzinger, J. and Barbour, R. S. (1999) 'Introduction: The challenge and promise of focus groups.' In R. S. Barbour and J. Kitzinger (eds) *Developing focus group research. Politics, theory and practice*, pp.1–20. London: Sage.

Kitzinger, J. and Farquhar, C. (1999) 'The analytical potential of "sensitive moments" in focus group discussions.' In R. S. Barbour and J. Kitzinger (eds) *Developing focus group research. Politics, theory and practice*, pp.156–172. London: Sage.

Krueger, R. A. (1993) 'Quality control in focus group research.' In D. L. Morgan (ed) *Successful Focus Groups: Advancing the State of the Art, 65–85.* London: Sage Publications.

Krueger, R.A. (1998) *Moderating Focus Groups.* Focus Group Kit, Volume 4. London: Sage.

Lam, J. and Beech, L. (1994) 'I'm sorry to go home'. The weekend break project: Consultation with users and their carers. Department of Psychology, St Helier NHS Trust, Sutton Hospital, Surrey.

Mason, J. (1996) Qualitative researching. London: Sage.

Merton, R. K., Fiske, M. and Kendall, P. L. (1956) The focused interview. Glencoe, Illinois: Free Press.

Michell, L. (1999) 'Combining focus groups and interviews: Telling how it is; telling how it feels.' In R. S. Barbour and J. Kitzinger (eds) Developing focus group research: Politics, theory and practice, pp.36–46. London: Sage.

Morgan, D. L. (1993) 'Future directions for focus groups.' In D. L. Morgan (ed) Successful focus groups: advancing the state of the art, pp.225–244. London: Sage.

Morgan, D. L. (1997) Focus groups as qualitative research. Second Edition. California: Sage Publications.

Morgan, D. L. and Krueger, R. A. (1993) 'When to use focus groups and why.' In D. L. Morgan (ed) Successful Focus Groups: Advancing the State of the Art, pp.3–19. London: Sage.

Oakley, A. (1981) 'Interviewing women: A contradiction in terms.' In H. Roberts (ed) Doing feminist research, pp.30–61. London: Routledge and Kegan Paul.

Qureshi, H., Patmore, C., Nicholas, E. and Bamford, C. (1998) 'Overview: Outcomes of social care for older people and carers.' Outcomes in Community Care Practice, Number 5. York: Social Policy Research Unit, University of York.

Schoenberg, N. E. and Ravdal, H. (2000) 'Using case studys in awareness and attitudinal research.' International Journal of Social Research Methodology 3, 1, 63–74.

Smith, M. W. (1995) 'Ethics in focus groups – a few concerns.' Qualitative Health Research 5, 4, 478–486.

Sperlinger, D. and McAuslane, L. (1993) 'I don't want you to think I'm ungrateful...but it doesn't satisfy what I want': A pilot study of the views of users of services for people with dementia in the London Borough of Sutton. Department of Psychology, St Helier NHS Trust, Sutton Hospital, Surrey.

Stewart, D. W. and Shamdasani, P. N. (1998) 'Focus group research: exploration and discovery.' In L. Bickman and D. J. Rog (eds) Handbook of Applied Social Research Methods, pp.505–526. London: Sage.

Stewart, J. (1996) 'Innovation in democratic practice in local government.' Policy and Politics 24, 1, 29–41.

Vaughn, S., Schumm, J. S. and Sinagub, J. (1996) Focus Group Interviews in Education and Psychology. London: Sage.

Yale, R. (1991) A guide to facilitating support groups for newly diagnosed Alzheimer's patients. Palo Alto, California: Alzheimer's Association.

Chapter Ten

'Nobody's ever asked how I felt'

Rebekah Pratt

Introduction

Interviewing people with dementia has become an increasingly important aspect of dementia research. Whilst the field has started to recognise the value of including people with dementia (Cotrell and Schulz 1993; Downs 1997) it is still learning how to conduct interviews in the most effective ways. There are many different ways to conduct interviews (Holloway and Jefferson 2000) but what is it about interviewing people with dementia that is different from interviewing other groups of people?

There are a number of issues that are particularly relevant to interviewing people with dementia. These issues relate to the nature of dementia and the impact of dementia on people's cognitive abilities. As social scientists we may lack useful knowledge about dementia, its causes, different types, symptoms and effects. It is this type of information that allows us to understand the way in which people with dementia may be different from other groups of people. Understanding these differences helps us as researchers to develop effective and appropriate ways of interviewing people with dementia.

This chapter will reflect on my experiences as a researcher working with people with early-stage dementia and will discuss some issues I faced in developing effective ways of interviewing. These issues do not relate to dementia exclusively, but are issues I felt were particularly relevant to the development of my own research practice. This includes the development of safe contexts, aspects of method, informed consent and developing reflective practice. This chapter will not provide all the answers, or a 'how to' guide on interviewing people with dementia. It will emphasise the factors every researcher can benefit from considering in the development of her or his style of interviewing.

My experience of the research[1] serves as a basis for this chapter. The research explored the effect of being told the diagnosis of dementia from the perspective of the person with dementia. This research aimed to address the gap of knowledge created by the exclusion of people with dementia from the debate on whether or not to disclose the diagnosis of dementia (Pratt and Wilkinson 2001). The study had three main objectives: to explore how people with dementia feel about the way in which they were told the diagnosis, to gain insight into the opportunities and limitations offered by an early diagnosis for the person with dementia, and to guide best practice in diagnosis disclosure. All quotes used in this chapter have been extracted from this research and all names used are pseudonyms.

Creating safe contexts

Applying the notion of safety to our research practice is an important part of working effectively with people with dementia. The term 'safety' is often used in relation to practitioner roles, where safety can be monitored and evaluated by considering individual practice. By adopting this notion of safety to research, and considering ourselves as practitioners of research, we can work in a way that is safe for people with dementia. This notion of safety is consistent with and has been influenced by both feminist (Riger 1992) and community psychology methodologies (Duckett and Fryer 1998). Both approaches relate to a number of values that aim to address the power inequality of the research relationship by developing empowering methods that contextualise the experience of research participants (Duckett and Pratt 2001; Wilkinson 1986). There are a number of key issues that relate to developing safe practice, such as the relationship with gatekeepers, carers, role ambiguity and dealing with distress.

Gatekeepers

We encounter a number of gatekeepers when negotiating access to people with dementia (such as doctors, community psychiatric nurses and support agencies). Much of the gatekeeping reflects the need for a vulnerable group of people to be cared for and protected. The gatekeepers are important in gaining access to people with dementia, and it is our job as researchers to show them that we will be 'safe' in our research practice of interviewing people with dementia (Pratt 2000). There may also be times when gatekeepers support views that people with dementia are not valid or reliable research participants. Involving them in the research process may provide an opportunity to challenge these views.

Often as researchers we perceive gatekeepers to be a barrier to research due to potentially paternalistic attitudes. These attitudes have been reflected in the practices of diagnosis disclosure (Vassilas 1999). However, gatekeepers can actually be useful resources when interviewing people with dementia. First they can be particularly important where there is either no carer or a poor relationship with a carer. Second, gatekeepers may potentially have the knowledge and relationship with the person with dementia to ensure we are being appropriate in our practice. They will often continue their relationship with the person with dementia well beyond the length of the research or interview relationship. This person then, when kept well informed of the research, can play a role in continuing to monitor the person with dementia's safety and understanding of the research process.

Key Points

Gatekeepers have a valid protective role.

Showing gatekeepers you are a safe practitioner adds accountability.

Involve gatekeepers as a resource to the research process and in supporting people with dementia into research.

The role of carers

Carers' attitudes have created barriers to increasing diagnosis disclosure rates (Maguire *et al.* 1996), raising concerns that carers may also be prohibitive to conducting research with people with dementia. Unlike gatekeepers, carers are mostly involved with the interviewee because of their relationship with that person, as partners or family members. This relationship may mean the carer has some potential insight into the person with dementia's experience. There are many occasions in which the relationship people with dementia have with carers may be strained. This may be the case if the person with dementia is trying to protect his/her family from the grief or pain he/she is experiencing (Gisser 1994). When there is a good relationship with the carer, the carer can actually be a useful collaborator in the research process.

If your interviewing style is interactive and allows carers to support the person with dementia during the interviews, you may find the carer can ask the person with dementia the questions in the best possible way. Carers may ask important questions you have not considered. This is particularly the case in open interviews, where the interviewing style is informal and conversational. The following extract is from an interview with Phil. Phil's wife was also present at this interview. During the interview she was quiet and not wanting to interrupt. During our conversation we started to discuss whether Phil could see any potential benefit if he had received an earlier diagnosis than he had been given; his wife asked if she could ask a question:

Phil's wife: Given that now we know that you've possibly had dementia for four or more years, would you have preferred to know four years ago, instead of spending the last four years thinking you had stress and depression?

Phil gave his wife's question careful consideration and gave the following answer:

Phil: That's a good one hen. As long as it's not progressing fast then I would like to know. If it's slow in

> progression then that's going to give me a bit more
> time.

Interviewing people with dementia with their carers may be a way to help the person feel more comfortable during the interview. Nevertheless it does change the nature of the interview. The ideal situation would be to conduct a number of interviews, some with carers present and some without. This scenario would allow the researcher to enjoy the benefits of the carer as a collaborator, to experience an observation of relationships, as well as having the value of individual interviews.

Key Points

Not all people with dementia and their carers have good relationships.

Carers can become valuable collaborators in the research process.

Combine interviews with and without carers if possible.

The Questioner Becomes the Questioned

Often in research we can assume the people we are interviewing know who we are and why we are there. We cannot make the same assumption when working with people experiencing short-term memory loss. If a person with dementia forgets who you are during the interview it is likely they may try to work out who you are.

Mary: What's your experience of people long term, people with Alzheimer's?

As you are there talking with them about their dementia it may be a reasonable assumption that you are medical staff or a social worker. This can mean you are asked questions that you cannot or should not answer. Before being placed in this situation you need to be clear about what questions you can and cannot answer.

Mary: And the thing is, is anybody halting Alzheimer's? Stopping it?

I asked people difficult questions and also had to deal with them asking me questions such as: 'How can you help me?', 'Is it right that this will never get better?', 'What is the difference between dementia and Alzheimer's?', 'Tell me honestly, am I any worse since you last visited?', 'How will it actually kill me?'.

Sarah: Is it true that this is terminal?

It is up to individual researchers to assess each situation when asked difficult questions. It is important to be honest with interviewees without providing information that is outside your knowledge base as a researcher. One way to approach this is to answer questions by reflecting the experiences of others to the person with dementia. Mary asked many difficult questions and often forgot why I was visiting her. It is important to deal with the questions as well as re-establishing why you are there. In Mary's case I answered her questions by using a positive reflective process of talking about the experiences of other interviewees.

Researcher: And do all of these people that know you, do they know about the Alzheimer's?

Mary: Yes, I've told every single one of them yes, I think it's important that they know and they are very sympathetic and very understanding, because I know I repeat myself, I keep on doing it, and thing, ooohh, but it's too late then, you've done it. Is this, I mean, how many other Alzheimer's people have you spoken to?

Researcher: I've spoken to another – people.

Mary: And does anything ring a bell with them?

Researcher: Yes.

Mary: Same sort of thing?

Researcher: Same sort of thing, same kinds of problems, yes.

Mary: Do they deal with them? Well I suppose nobody deals with their problems in exactly the same way, or find a way round it.

Researcher: What I have found is that everyone seems to be good at finding a really positive way to not let it get them down – which sounds the same as you?

Mary: I would agree with that yes, because I do wonder about people, how they reacted to a situation like this, because it's, it's pretty sick making when you think about it you know. To lose your memory, it's such an important part of your life.

Re-establishing who you are and why you are there is an important part of being sure you have informed consent for the interview. Clarifying your role helps in maximising informed consent.

Key Points

Be prepared for difficult questions.

Be aware that role ambiguity can easily happen.

Find ways both to address the questions and re-establish why you are there.

Dealing with distress

An important part of creating safe contexts is to consider ways in which we can deal with potentially distressing situations. I was interviewing people about their experience of receiving a diagnosis of dementia. This was a topic that was potentially very distressing and indeed it was an emotional topic to discuss for many participants (Pratt and Wilkinson 2001). It was important to develop strategies for handling distress prior to the interviews.

The strategies I engaged in to minimise their distress included active listening and offering breaks from the interview. I also ensured there was time and space for people to talk through their distress if they wanted to.

The 'right' strategy is one that responds to the needs of the person during the interview. I was committed to making the interview process as positive for participants as possible. I spent time at the end of the interview reflecting back to people the positive approaches they had described using to deal with their dementia.

Peter was one person who was particularly distressed during interviewing. It was made very clear to me by the referring agency that Peter was experiencing distress, however he also felt it was very important to talk about his views on diagnosis. The interview was difficult for Peter as he was very upset by his diagnosis of dementia.

Researcher:	Do you ever wish you'd not been told that?
Peter:	No, no I couldn't have gone on for all these years without knowing what it was.
Researcher:	So the hardness of dealing with it hasn't been a good enough reason not to know?
Peter:	No (whisper) no. No I had to know.

I felt it was important to listen to Peter for as long as he wanted to talk and to provide the opportunity for him to express his feelings. I also offered to terminate the interview at points and when he was ready we did terminate it. Terminating the interview meant staying with Peter until he was feeling calmer. This created time to have conversation about non-distressing topics, including positive reflection to Peter about his coping strategies.

Peter was provided further support from the gatekeepers who arranged our initial contact. The negotiations with the agencies who referred people with dementia to the study meant that there would be follow-up with people if they did become distressed. In this example it was a combination of my own strategies and the good relationships I had negotiated with the gatekeepers around Peter that contributed to his safety as an interviewee.

Key Points

Find strategies to deal with distress during interviews, including ways to end the interview.

Distress does not necessarily mean the interview needs to be stopped.

People may want to talk through their distress.

Informed consent

Where much research relies on participants to have the competency required to provide informed consent, the assessment of what level of competency people with dementia have is often uncertain. Developing a way to consider competency that is context-relevant is important (Collopy 1988). In the context of social research it is important to consider how competent a person is to consent to discuss their feelings and experiences. A number of studies have established that people with dementia are competent to consent to this (Husband 1999; Robinson Ekman and Wahlund 1998; Sabat 1994).

There are a number of issues relating to informed consent and the ethics of working with a 'vulnerable' group. There is no way to guarantee 100 per cent informed consent when working with people with dementia. In the area of dementia research the limitations of short-term memory require researchers to consider carefully how to engage in a process of maximising informed consent. This involves using the relationships with gatekeepers and carers to provide us with reassurances about how well the person with dementia understands the research and how happy they are to consent to take part in the research. It also requires viewing informed consent as a process that happens over time and not just something that is checked at one point only (Pratt and Wilkinson 2001).

There are positive benefits to involving key people in the consent process, as they may be needed to help remind the person with dementia about the research, both in content and in the arrangements for interviewing.

One issue that is particular to the area of dementia research is how you present the research project, for example do you describe your research as being about dementia? There is always a possibility that people are not informed about their diagnosis or, if they have been informed, may have forgotten. Again, the relationship with other key people can be useful for ascertaining exactly what information a person with dementia has about his/her diagnosis, if indeed they know it at all. Taking time to talk with interviewees about the symptoms of dementia before introducing questions about the diagnosis is important. Ways to talk about symptoms can be to discuss difficulties in finding the right words, forgetfulness, name recall, money handling and obsessive behaviour.

It is also useful to be aware of the way in which people can use metaphor to describe their experiences of dementia. The example of Harry illustrates this well. Harry would talk about his feeling of loss and grief by not only talking about his diagnosis of dementia but also by describing his feelings about his hearing loss and the death of his son (Pratt and Wilkinson 2001, p.31).

It is useful to develop a protocol to ensure you do not accidentally disclose the diagnosis inappropriately. It may include:

1. Checking with all key people about the individual's knowledge of his/her diagnosis.

2. Not mentioning the diagnosis of dementia until the person with dementia does.

3. Finding safe ways to introduce talk about dementia symptoms.

4. Prioritising safety and avoiding accidental diagnosis disclosure above informed consent.

5. Informing key people of your protocols.

When I interviewed Harry the protocols I used to avoid accidental disclosure of diagnosis worked well. On my first visit to Harry he was extremely articulate about his experiences of having dementia. He also very strongly advocated that people should be told when they have dementia. On our second conversation three months later I was expecting an equally articulate Harry. However his dementia had worsened to the point where our conversation didn't specifically cover dementia at all. This was because Harry had mostly forgotten that he had dementia. Following the protocol meant I would not mention the diagnosis of dementia until Harry mentioned it first. In this case that helped to maintain a safe environment for Harry to be interviewed in.

Key Points

Informed consent needs to be viewed as a process of checking and rechecking.

Use key people to increase your confidence in the person with dementia's consent.

Develop protocols to avoid accidental disclosure.

Matters of method

Research methodology itself can be a barrier to the inclusion of people with dementia into research. Positivist views of validity and reliability of participants can be reflected in setting inclusion criteria that may be unnecessarily restrictive. An example of this is the use of Mini Mental State Examination (MMSE) scores to determine if participants will be included in research, despite the fact that these scores do not necessarily indicate the ability of a person with dementia to talk about his/her life, experiences or needs (Pratt and Wilkinson 2001). Challenging methodology is an important part of encouraging research to be more inclusive of people with dementia.

People with dementia may have difficulty recalling certain types of information in an interview setting. By designing methods that focus on the strengths of participants' abilities, some of these issues can be overcome. Challenging the need and method of gathering baseline details about participants in research is important. Whilst these are useful for describing the group of people interviewed, these questions can sometimes be the most difficult in an interview with a person with dementia due to the reliance on short-term memory recall. An example of this is if you ask a participant their age. It can be very difficult for people with dementia to remember their age, however it may be easier for them to recall their date of birth. It is important to question the need for each baseline detail you collect, and then to find creative ways that do not rely on short-term memory to obtain the information.

Information that relies on the recollection of dates or the sequence of events may also be difficult to recall. It is important to consider what type of information you really require as a researcher. People with dementia talk with great consistency about their feelings or experiences; the validity of their responses are not lessened by the difficulty they may have in describing when they had certain experiences (Pratt and Wilkinson 2001).

Key Points

Focus on abilities rather than deficits during interviewing by asking about feelings and experiences rather than the recollection of 'facts'.

Challenge methods to be more inclusive of people with dementia.

Allowing time

One particular lesson I learned whilst interviewing people with dementia was the importance of time. One person to teach me this was Mary. On my first visit with Mary she presented as having fairly moderate dementia, and most of our interview was dominated by her reminiscing about her life. I arranged to visit Mary on a second occasion and was not expecting to get any information from her about how she felt about her diagnosis experience. The lesson Mary taught me was not to judge a person with dementia on any one point in time. Our second conversation was extremely relevant and she was able to talk with increased clarity and focus about her dementia. People with dementia have good days and bad days, they may experience changes over time and they may take time to open up to you (Pratt and Wilkinson 2001). Engaging in multiple interviews over time is extremely valuable. They allow you to observe and understand the context of each individual you interview. This is very useful information to help the researcher in understanding and interpreting meaning from the interview interactions.

Rapport can be developed in subsequent interviews, sometimes improving the content of the interview. In this project, most of the participants did not remember the interviewer or the first interview. Despite this, rapport was increased in the second interview. This could be attributed to a number of reasons, one being the good days and bad days people have. Interviewing on two occasions provided an increased opportunity to talk to people on the good days. The interviewer is able to conduct the interview building on the knowledge of the participant gained from the first interview, assisting the interviewer in knowing what issues to explore with each person. The increased skills and comfort of the interviewer with each participant may also have been a factor in why the second interview was often more informative (Pratt and Wilkinson 2001).

Key Points

There are great benefits to allowing more time.

People with dementia have good and bad days.

You can build rapport with people with dementia over time.

Developing reflective practice

A key to working effectively with people with dementia is to develop a reflective style of practice. This allows a researcher to consider how his/her values can impact on the research interaction (Wilkinson 1986). This is important for the development of appropriate methods, particularly when working with a group of people whose experiences you do not share. This reflection may help a researcher understand how his/her perspective may differ from the research participant (Riger 1992), which in turn can help identify appropriate methods and approaches to analysis.

There are several key aspects that may help in developing this style of working, such as supervision and considering interviewer safety.

Supervision

Developing reflective practice can be difficult to do in isolation. Seeking supervision from someone who has his/her own experiences and skills to help you develop your practice can assist it. A task you can ensure that you do, whether you are able to access supervision or not, is to make detailed field notes about your experiences and your own responses to interviewing for future reflection.

Supervision allows you as a researcher to consider the questions that may arise during the process of doing research. Formalising time when you can deal with these questions through supervision can be very helpful. It can also provide support for you as a researcher in tackling difficult subjects with interviewees in the most appropriate way.

One of the most valuable aspects of supervision is its use as a way to process your own emotional responses to the research and to consider your own safety as an interviewer. This was particularly highlighted to me when I talked to Sarah. Sarah was one of the younger participants in the dementia study. On my first visit, Sarah talked very openly about her shock and grief. She also had a fantastic sense of humour and we got on very well. It was one of the first times she had been able to talk about her feelings about receiving her diagnosis.

Sarah: Nobody's ever asked how I felt.

On the second visit three months later, Sarah had visibly declined. She had been trying anti-dementia medication but it was not having any effect. Sarah had also just learnt that Alzheimer's could be considered a terminal illness (you don't necessarily die from Alzheimer's, but it does decrease your life span). Sarah's husband also sat in on the second interview. It was clear that they had a tremendous amount of love for each other and their despair and grief about the Alzheimer's disease was immense.

Despite having listened to a number of different stories and witnessed different people's grief I was particularly affected by Sarah's story. It was through talking with other people who were experienced at working with issues of dying and grief that I was able to process my own sense of grief for Sarah and her family. Dealing with your own emotional responses is important to developing your practice as an interviewer. It is important to be emotionally present when interviewing people; it is a key part of interaction that happens in research. It is also a vital aspect of being present as a genuine person and not just a researcher. Through supervision you can identify and work on the issues, such as grief, that you face as a researcher.

Key Points

Supervision can be a very useful tool for developing practice.

Developing understanding of a discipline of interest can be a useful part of supervision.

It is important to consider your emotional responses to develop safe practices.

Interviewee safety

Researchers are involved in people's lives for very short periods of time. During this time we engage in an experience of talking with a person about what are often difficult issues. Then researchers leave the interviewing relationship to carry on with tasks of data preparation and analysis. But what happens to the person we have just taken through a process of discussing difficult issues? How do we know that we as researchers have not left a mess behind us?

A key factor in ensuring the safety of the people we interview is to use the multitude of relationships we negotiate in accessing people to interview. This means seeing gatekeepers and carers as a potentially important part of ensuring the safety of the interviewee. This is not to say that as researchers we pass on responsibility to these people; rather, we can work alongside them. Gatekeepers and carers know the person we interview far better than we do, and are likely to have an on-going relationship with them, potentially increasing accountability and support.

One way to check on the safety of people you interview is to build a reflective question into the interview about the interview process, or in other words, ask people how it is for them to talk about their experiences. This is a good way to gather information about your practice, both by getting indications that you are doing the right things and information about how to improve safety. In the case of Mary, she validated my practice as both suiting her and being beneficial.

Researcher: How have you found it to be able to talk to somebody about it, has it been okay to chat?

Mary: It's been absolute bliss because other people don't understand, and sometimes you get the sense that they feel uncomfortable with you, you know, not that you're a foreign being exactly, but that Alzheimer's sort of marks you off in a way. It's lovely because you don't make me feel like that at all.

In the case of Harry, he used that time to reflect on how difficult it can be to talk about his dementia. He also provided a great suggestion that we take a break from the hard issues and talk about something more cheerful for him. This checking-in with Harry opened an opportunity to conduct the interview in the safest way for him.

Harry: It worries me in that I think I'll die earlier than I should, because that's a notion I've got in my head, you know, but that's no big deal. I'll tell you something jolly.

Researcher: Yeah.

Harry: I was the first, the last person in the – .

Researcher: You were the last one?

Harry: Yeah, the very last one and I can talk, I'm only mentioning that because I've come to a sort of a hole there in what I was saying that I just wanted to talk about something else for a few minutes.

Key Points

Use the relationships with gatekeepers and carers to increase safety.

Check on interviewee safety by asking him/her about how it is for him/her.

Reflect on your own practice.

Concluding thoughts

This chapter was written to share some of my experiences of interviewing people with dementia with other researchers. There are several themes that emerge from the chapter. The first of these is the importance of relationships both with the person with dementia and those around him/her. These relationships are important and can offer potential routes to accountability and to support interviewees.

The concepts of safe and reflective practice are also important. Both of these are extremely useful tools for finding effective ways to interview people with dementia. Often these concepts are hidden in the research, the parts we don't share with colleagues and the academic world, particularly reflections on our emotional responses. Addressing safe and reflective practice will help you develop the skills you need as a researcher to deal with difficult issues.

A last theme of the chapter is the need for us to work in ways that respect the differences there might be between people with dementia and ourselves. This respect demands flexibility in our approaches and a need for us to be critical as researchers about what practices and methods achieve that respect.

Note

1   Rebekah Pratt was the researcher on a project entitled 'Sharing the diagnosis: the perspectives of people with a diagnosis of dementia' conducted with Dr Heather Wilkinson and funded by The Mental Health Foundation (United Kingdom).

References

Collopy, B. (1988) 'Autonomy in long term care: Some crucial distinctions.' *Gerontologist* 28, 10–18.

Cotrell, V. and Schulz, R. (1993) 'The perspective of the person with Alzheimer's Disease: A neglected dimension of dementia research.' *Gerontologist 33*, 205–211.

Downs, M. (1997) 'The emergence of the person in dementia research.' *Ageing and Society 17*, 597–607.

Duckett, P. and Fryer, D. (1998) 'Developing empowering research practices with people who have learning disabilities.' *Journal of Community and Applied Social Psychology 8*, 57–65.

Duckett, P. and Pratt, R. (2001) 'The researched opinions on research: Visually impaired people and visual impairment research.' *Disability and Society.*

Gisser, N. (1994) 'Keeping a focus on the quality of life.' *Alzheimer Association Cleveland Area Chapter* July 10–14.

Holloway, W. and Jefferson, T. (2000) *Doing Qualitative Research Differently.* London: Sage Publications.

Husband, H. J. (1999) 'The psychological consequences of learning a diagnosis of dementia: Three case examples.' *Aging and Mental Health 3*, 2, 179–183.

Maguire, C. P., Kirby, M., Wen, R., Coakley, D., Lawlor, B. A. and O'Neill, D. (1996) 'Family members' attitudes towards telling the patient with AD their diagnosis.' *BMJ 313*, 529–530.

Pratt, R. (2000) *'Involving the person with dementia into research.'* Involving People with Dementia into Research Symposium. Centre for Social Research on Dementia, University of Stirling.

Pratt, R. and Wilkinson, H. (2001) *No Diagnosis Has to be Your Whole Life: The effect of being told the diagnosis of dementia from the perspective of the person with dementia. Final Report to the Mental Health Foundation.* London: Mental Health Foundation.

Riger, S. (1992) 'Epistemological debates, feminist voices.' *American Psychologist* June, 730–740

Robinson, P., Ekman, S. L. and Wahlund, L. O. (1998) 'Unsettled, Uncertain and Striving to understand: Toward an understanding of the situation of persons with suspected dementia.' *International Journal of Aging and Human Development 47*, 2, 143–161.

Sabat, S. (1994) 'Recognising and working with remaining abilities: Toward improving the care of Alzheimer's disease sufferers.' *The American Journal of Alzheimer's Care and Related Disorders Research 8*, 16.

Vassilas, C. (1999) 'How often do GPs tell people with dementia the truth about their diagnosis?' *Alzheimer's Disease Society*, February.

Wilkinson, S. (1986) 'Sighting possibilities: Diversity and commonality in feminist research'. In S. Wilkinson (ed.) *Feminist social psychology: Developing theory and practice.* Buckingham: Open University Press.

Chapter 11

Don't leave me hanging on the telephone
Interviews with people with dementia using the telephone

Anne Mason and Heather Wilkinson

Introduction

Eliciting user perspectives is an explicit and accepted aim within health and social care practice (NHS and Community Care Act 1990; Patients Charter 1998) and within legal reforms (Adults with Incapacity (Scotland) Act – see Scottish Executive 2000). People with dementia represent a large number of these users. It is estimated that the number of people with dementia in the UK will have increased to 855,000 by the year 2020 (Department of Health 1997). Cultural constructs of disability and disabling values and attitudes discriminate and exclude 'disabled' people from expressing their views and experiences (Goldsmith 1996; Priestley 1999). The ability of the person with dementia to express their views has been ignored due to predominant interest in the disease process (Cotrell and Schulz 1993). Ideological shifts away from this traditional medical model of health toward a psycho-social understanding have assisted in progressing toward the recognition that people with dementia, who may well have some difficulties with cognition, have an important contribution to make toward the development of social policies and services.

The aim of the present chapter is to examine critically the feasibility of using the telephone as a method to ascertain the views of people with dementia. This will be done by drawing from a recent research project to explore the use of the Scottish legal system by people with dementia (Mason and Wilkinson 2001). The ethos of involving people with dementia in the research process was guided by the principle of user involvement and the principles underpinning the Adults with Incapacity (Scotland) Act (Scottish Executive 2000).[1] The potential benefits and limitations of using the telephone with people who have dementia, the skills required for telephone interviewing, ethical issues, the interview process and the challenge this presents to researchers will be explored.

In commercial research the telephone interview has become increasingly popular, especially in order to engage large numbers of individuals at low cost whilst avoiding the low participation figures common in postal surveys. There are also examples of telephone interviews being used successfully with vulnerable groups such as people with depression (Aneshensel *et al.* 1982); for surveying diagnoses of alcoholism (Slutske *et al.* 1998); for assessing bi-polar disorders (Revicki *et al.* 1997); and for providing psychotherapy by telephone (McLaren 1992). In the field of dementia there are some examples of using the telephone to support and build the skills of family carers (Davis 1998). Other types of communication such as computer assisted technology used to support and/or offer therapeutic interventions for users and carers are also reported in the literature (Hanson, Tetley and Shewan 2000; Peiris, Alm and Gregor 1995).

More recently there are examples of research using the telephone specifically with older people and in attempts to assess cognitive status (Barak, Macdonald and Levy 1998; Brandt, Spencer and Folstein 1988). Brandt *et al.* (1988) developed a cognitive screening test for administration by telephone based on a study of 100 people with Alzheimer's disease (AD). The test was successful at discriminating people with even mild AD from healthy controls.

However, as a method for collecting both quantitative and qualitative data focusing on personal experiences and views, the telephone had not been tested with people with dementia. There was some evidence that people with dementia did still use the telephone and a recent study of a dementia helpline found that a significant proportion of callers were people with dementia (Keady *et al.* 1999).

For the purpose of this study the telephone interview method was chosen for two main reasons. First, to gather information from a larger number of participants in a cost-effective manner, and second, to explore the use of the telephone as a way of gathering the views of people with dementia. Considering the feasibility of interviewing people with dementia by telephone requires a critical examination of the following questions:

> What is different about the person with dementia that might cause them difficulty if being interviewed by telephone?

> Does the telephone have any advantages that can help with the particular problems experienced by the person with dementia?

> What are its failings?

> What are the necessary skills?

> What can be achieved? What cannot be achieved?

The following debate offers insight into answering these questions, drawn from telephone interviews with 26 people with dementia.

Background to the study

The study aimed to examine the use of the legal system by people with dementia, living in Scotland.[2] Four geographical areas were chosen as a representation of the geographical divides of Scotland. The aims of the study were to:

1. describe the characteristics of people with dementia who are users and non-users of the Scottish legal system

2. identify what facilitates or hinders the uptake of the Scottish legal system by people with dementia

3. examine the feasibility of interviewing people with dementia by telephone.

Pilot study

The sensitive nature of the study, combined with the use of the telephone, was correctly raised as an ethical issue. These ethical dilemmas required the researchers to approach this study with caution and the pilot study was an essential beginning.

It was crucial to identify a safe, protected and practical protocol that would allow the researchers access to people with dementia living within their communities. The pilot phase was carried out to test the effectiveness of:

>	assessment for inclusion into the study

>	the recruitment and sampling strategy

>	the interview process

>	validity and reliability issues

>	consent procedures

>	telephone interviewing.

The initial recruitment method for the sample was through general practitioners (GPs) and the extended health team. Eventually, community psychiatric nurses (CPNs) were identified as key health professionals. Advantages to this route included the CPN's knowledge of the person. They were also in a position to consider the wider family network and the presence of any key carer. The CPN route to recruitment was an important finding during the pilot stage and it was found to be not only effective but also 'safe' for the patient, the carer and the researcher. Safety is a key issue in terms of access to people and in gaining their consent. The procedures followed by the CPNs meant an emphasis was placed on safeguarding the person's identity prior to consent, and ensured that the cognitive processes required to make a decision to participate or not were supported, by offering step-by-step information about participation, independent from the researcher. The researcher was assured of the continuous relationship between the respondent and the CPN post interview. CPNs made clinical judgements about the patient's capacity to be involved using the following criteria:

Has the person been informed of their diagnosis?

Does the person still use a telephone regularly?

Is the person's emotional state stable?

Does the person have the cognitive capacity and memory to contribute verbally to a conversation and to discuss daily living issues?

Can the person indicate verbally their understanding of the consent form?

Meetings were arranged with CPNs to explain the study, the inclusion criteria, the ethical agreements, the purpose of the study, a sample of the types of questions and style of interview. The background and skills of the researcher was also raised at these meetings. It was an opportunity for CPNs to raise concerns, similar to those already expressed by the ethics committees.

The recruitment procedures had a direct effect on the sample. The initial research design anticipated a random stratified sample of people with dementia. It became apparent during the pilot and from a parallel study (Pratt and Wilkinson 2001) that accessing people with dementia was problematic due to the restraints of professional practices and that a random sample was unrealistic. The final sample was derived from CPNs caseloads and was entirely dependent on their clinical judgement.

The consent form was designed specifically for this client group. Bjorn et al. (1999) suggest ways in which written information to research subjects can be improved: these include cognitive understanding of the subject matter. These were incorporated into the design and examined by the local Alzheimers' Scotland Action on Dementia (ASAD) organisation in Inverness.

The pilot also allowed the researchers to test the interview method, the interview schedule and the skills required by the researcher, to enable the person with dementia to engage successfully in a telephone interview. The participants were encouraged to express their feelings about being interviewed by telephone. This information was carefully examined by the researchers and the ethical committees prior to commencing the main study. The small number of respondents interviewed by telephone during the pilot expressed a positive and enjoyable experience. The interview method and schedule were developed with the help of the respondents. The final approach offered some structure to the interview but encouraged the person to discuss his/her position from his/her own social and family contexts. The interviewer was able to reflect on the interview process to identify what skills were required to support the person through each stage of the interview process.

The reliability and validity of the research methods were considered at the pilot stage. The content validity of the instrument was examined by a variety of professional health clinicians, solicitors, voluntary organisations, carers, and one person with dementia. The interview method, schedule and cognitive capacity of the respondents were critically examined. The style of the interview developed and became more flexible to the needs of the respondents to help them engage productively and meaningfully within the interview.

The use of the telephone was of considerable interest at the pilot stage. Assessment of respondents' ability to use the phone was accurate. All respondents appeared at ease with the telephone. It was evident that respondents enjoyed the experience and the opportunity for the conversation.

One of the key results of the pilot study was the refocusing of the approach from quantitative to a more qualitative methodology. The underlying principles of the Adults with Incapacity (Scotland) Act (2000) emphasise a person-centred focus, and the pilot study indicated that a breadth and depth of rich data could be gathered from people with dementia.

The main study

Interviewing has been described by Mishler (1986) as a 'jointly constructed discourse between the respondent and interviewer that promotes a regard for the social and personal context of the respondent as part of this process' (p.52). Mishler argues that the interview should facilitate a collaborative and participatory role for the respondent with the aim to empower.

Transferring the notion of empowerment from an ideological intent into practice presents professional challenges across disciplines and at all levels.

The challenge of including people with dementia within the present research study and interviewing by telephone was multifarious. The process of inclusion had to be ethically sound. Traditional research and health paradigms were contested. Discriminatory practices were questioned. The ability of people with dementia to participate, the validity of their responses, people's rights to their own diagnostic information, the interview process and qualitative research methodology were constant dilemmas during the course of this study. The protocol for accessing and including people with dementia, the skills of the interviewer and the interview process were critically detailed at every stage of the research process. The development of an interview process that promoted and respected the individual's perspective was the primary reason for overcoming moral, philosophical and methodological arguments for not including the views and experiences of people with dementia. Two key texts (Mishler 1986; Rosenfield 1997) have helped guide this process. The following skill categories have been adapted from Rosenfield's chapter on 'Skills and Attitudes' (chapter 2), extending the debate to include the research interview and contextualising these skills in relation to working with people who have dementia.

Welcoming the participant to the interview

Rosenfield divides the interview process into various stages and suggests that good relationships can be quickly established by telephone when welcoming the person. This was experienced within the present study, with extended invitations from respondents to 'call in'. Receiving consent from a respondent, with his/her telephone number, was the first step in giving the researcher permission to contact him/her. The initial phone call was to introduce the researcher and the study, to ascertain that consent was still forthcoming and to arrange an interview time convenient to the person. The researcher was prepared to interview on this first call but did not assume that this initial contact was convenient or that the person would remember the consent form or detail about the study.

These first moments with the participant were crucial to the interview process. The researcher conveyed a non-threatening and respectful manner. Ascertaining the person's memory of consent required sensitivity. The first few words, and that sentences were adapted to prevent alienating the person. Rosenfield suggests that the person does not hear the first few words and important information can be relayed once a rapport has been established. Hence the researcher's tone of voice was considered more important at this point. The general approach was informal and purpose-ful.

Various types of reactions occurred at this stage. Some people immedi-ately interceded claiming recognition of the project. Others were a little more hesitant until the name of their CPN was introduced to the conversa-tion as a memory trigger. Their voices became more relaxed and friendly at this point. Several could not recall signing the consent or admitted to a vague recollection. However, this was a familiar experience for respon-dents who were accustomed to such difficulties and openly acknowledged these to the researcher. It was an everyday occurrence for them. The most prominent recall problem was from a woman who could not remember signing the consent form. Mary appeared very au fait with the conversa-tion and suggested further contact by telephone an hour later when it would be more convenient. The second phone call was met with no recall of the first conversation but again this respondent clearly understood the present conversation and purpose of the call, although could not retain this within her memory.

Once consent had been confirmed with respondents and the researcher was confident that it was a convenient time for the person to talk, the researcher proceeded with the interview. It was necessary to verbally check the person's level of comfort and privacy. The researcher again reminded the person that the interview could be stopped at any time. Some people volunteered feelings of self-doubt about the interview at this stage. The researcher described the format, explaining that there were some specific (demographic) questions but most of the time was to chat about what it was like to have some 'memory difficulties'. The flexibility of the interview was emphasised, indicating that there were questions that could be used to guide the conversation. Most people implied that they were willing just to see how the interview progressed. One man explained that he was worried that he 'might dry up'. Such openness at an early stage in the interview was extremely helpful to understanding his anxieties and possible cognitive problems that might arise during the course of the interview.

Structure of interview

The researcher decided to begin with demographic questions. The reason for the chosen structure was to help the person feel confident in his/her ability to answer. During the pilot, these questions were answered with ease and the person's tone of voice seemed to settle and become lighter and less hesitant as he/she moved through them. It had the advantage of allowing the respondent to get used to the researcher's voice and get a sense of the researcher as a person. Most people answered the specific questions at the beginning prior to the more open and less structured part of the interview. A few initiated their own dialogue fairly quickly, often triggered by one of the demographic questions. Demographic detail was collected at the end of the interview in such instances.

Responses helped the researcher to form a gradual picture of the person such as their living arrangements and relationships. This itself led into a more natural and exploratory part of the interview in which questions were not presented unexpectedly. The researcher attempted to restructure the relationship with the respondent in a way that would facilitate an empowering experience, shifting the balance of power away from the researcher. However, there was also a need to be sensitive to the expectations and abilities of the interviewee. Some responded well to this open approach to the interview and 'told' their story from diagnosis to the present day in a semi-structured way. Others were more comfortable with a structured approach to the interview and sought guidance from the researcher as to the direction and flow of the interview. This flexible and responsive approach was essential to the outcomes of the interview.

Core skills required for telephone interviewing

Rosenfield makes the important distinction between counselling by telephone and using counselling skills over the telephone. She argues that the skills necessary to develop the therapeutic relationship required for counselling by telephone can be used in more one-off communications with people looking for a range of help through the various helplines available today. She identifies several common categories for working with people by telephone including information giving, advice giving, advocacy, support, befriending and counselling. Opposition to using the telephone for counselling interviewing is based on the assumption that it is less effective than a face-to-face encounter. It has also been portrayed as a less effective research method if the interviewer is unknown to the respondent (Polit and Hungler 1999). Rosenfield suggests part of this unease to recognise the telephone as an effective communication medium might be more to do with the relinquishing of power. The respondent can terminate the call in one quick action. She points out that the development of standards (National Vocational Qualifications) have helped to endorse the use of the telephone and guides the reader to the *Guidelines for Good Practice in Telephone Work* (Telephone Helplines Association 1993).

Although the research interview is neither a counselling situation nor a helpline, the skills described by Rosenfield are crucial to methods used within this study. The client group under discussion, that is, those people who have been given a diagnosis of dementia, are potentially vulnerable. Their ability to make themselves understood and to comprehend the focus of the interview is likely to be impaired to some extent due to the impact of the dementia on their cognition. In order to support the person who has problems with their cognition and associated self-esteem issues (Kitwood and Bredin 1992) the researcher needs to help the person to engage in the interview successfully.

Counselling and interpersonal skills are a necessary part of this process. Empathy is considered a key component of such skills (Kalisch 1971; Mason 1990; Reynolds 1986). Empathy is exhibited when certain aspects of perception, cognition, feeling and behaviour are brought together (La Monica 1981). Hence, skills such as listening attentively to the content and emotion offered during interviews, and providing warmth and genuineness, promote an environment that is non-threatening. Such skills reinforce the idea of a joint discourse where the interviewer and interviewee together produce a final account of experiences that is meaningful to the person being interviewed. Such discourse is considered central to shifting the attention away from the research 'problem' and more toward the respondent's 'problems'. This paradigm shift, recommended by Mishler (1986), respects the respondent's view of the world, and is attentive and potentially empowering. This chapter describes the steps that are taken to ensure the respondent is the predominate agent within the interview process, with consideration given to their human rights, their vulnerability and abilities. The skills used during telephone interviews with people with dementia are detailed here to demonstrate the level of discourse achieved.

Listening and responding skills

Listening is the most essential skill when using the telephone (Rosenfield 1997). In this study the researcher and respondent relied totally on the spoken word, the content, and how it was presented. The interviewer needed to 'be there' for the person. The use of verbal gesturing was exaggerated on the telephone to ensure a sense of presence, encouragement and interest. The researcher worked at providing energy and animation through the spoken word. Yet, the invitation to expand or clarify issues was tentative, to ensure that the respondent did not feel pressured.

The researcher had a heightened awareness and concentration at all times during the telephone interview. The skills needed for person-centred interviewing whether face to face or by telephone are basically the same, but the emphasis is different. There was a need to be more explicit to compensate for the lack of visual aids. The researcher was attentive to:

emotional content

personal attributes

cognitive difficulties

terminology

willingness to participate

openness and confidentiality

personal values.

Changes in a person's communication often created uncertainty for the researcher about how the respondent was coping with the interview and these were sometimes shared with the respondent. However, this had to be a careful and calculated consideration. The need to share was weighed against the danger of alienating the respondent or causing additional stress. Appropriate sharing led to a more relaxed and open discussion. The following accounts illustrate the attention given to these aspects of communication.

EMOTIONAL CONTENT

One respondent had a very shaky voice as if it would break at any moment. This affected the researcher's style of communication. Lack of visual aids made it more difficult to ascertain how comfortable the respondent was with the interview. The researcher chose to share this uncertainty with the respondent. The respondent had been discussing a physical ailment that was causing her more concern than her memory difficulties. The researcher shared this understanding with her prior to asking her,

Researcher: It is difficult not being beside you. I hear some upset in your voice, and wonder how you are feeling just now. … Do you want to continue…?

Respondent: Oh, I know what you mean. My voice is like this all the time. I call it my sexy voice. I don't mind talking!

If this dilemma had not been shared the interview might have progressed differently and the researcher might have made incorrect assumptions about the respondent's experiences and abilities.

PERSONAL ATTRIBUTES

Listening and responding to personal attributes were fundamental to the aims of the study. They contributed to how the researcher approached the respondent's difficulties. They also provided clues for the researcher as to what the respondent might cope with during the interview. It could be argued that such clues were more objective than those picked up from a face-to-face interview. There was no opportunity to prejudge a respondent from his/her living conditions or appearance. The only potential bias came from the respondent's 'voice'.

During the course of an interview with a female respondent, it became apparent that she was the type of person who was able to face things, was insightful to her cognitive difficulties and welcomed some honest discussion. The researcher was attentive to such attributes that in turn encouraged this respondent to expand more deeply on some of her experiences.

Respondent: They (meaning the family) don't really want to know, Anne. It's not that they don't care, it's their way of dealing with it. They say things like, 'oh there is nothing wrong with you'. They used to torment me and say, 'oh you've forgotten again'. But since the diagnosis they don't do that anymore. I miss that. I don't want them to treat me differently.

It seemed important to this woman that the bantering continued and was familiar to her. The researcher respected this and was able to explore issues with her more confidently.

COGNITIVE DIFFICULTIES

Several people did have difficulty expressing themselves due to their cognitive difficulties. This would have been a problem for them whether the interview had been conducted by telephone or face to face. The additional difficulty over the telephone was in ascertaining how the respondent was coping with such difficulties. These were portrayed as a vagueness and an inability to expand or discuss. Some were insightful about their difficulties and requested that the researcher spoke to their carer (usually a family member) for further elaboration or clarification. Others were more guarded.

Respondent: That is something I am not sure about. I think I did mention it [memory difficulties] in the passing to a very nice Doctor... Can't really remember, Anne. I don't recall her telling me anything.

This difficulty in recall was fairly constant during this interview. The researcher felt this respondent needed more guidance and structure through the interview and was sensitive to the amount of questions asked that might have a similar reply. The respondent did not appear troubled by this difficulty with recall and volunteered at the closing of the interview:

Respondent: I don't mind the phone. You are very understanding, Anne. I really enjoyed the chat.

Although invited to discuss what it was like to have memory difficulties, some respondents had difficulty with open questions and the interview progressed in a more structured question-and-answer style. It is likely that the respondent's cognitive abilities might cause difficulties with elaboration, due to problems with recall. Yet, interviewing people who have no cognitive difficulties will also produce a diversity of depth and ability to cope with the interview. Trust, power issues, skills of the researcher, personalities, past experience, and education are just some of the barriers experienced during interviews. The following respondent demonstrated difficulties with her recall, but the content of her answers also indicated an attempt to be in control and to present as 'normal':

Respondent: It is forgetfulness. My short-term memory. I am no worse than I was. I pay them (bills) myself. I am not in any debt.

This is a good example of where counselling skills are used in a one-off session to gather an empathic understanding of the person but not to offer counselling. The aim of the interview is different. It was not appropriate or timely to pursue possible self-esteem and identity issues that were being conveyed by this respondent. The researcher detected some cognitive problems which the respondent seemed guarded about, and responded to these by selecting the type of questions, the structure and depth of the interview, that seemed most suited to this respondent. The researcher felt the respondent needed the pressure taken off and a more passive approach was adopted due to the singular nature of the interview.

TERMINOLOGY

Terminology was raised as a major ethical concern during this study. Although respondents invited into this study were required to know their diagnosis, the terms used to describe their dementia were unknown. The researcher used the term 'memory difficulties' unless the respondent used other descriptions. This reduced the danger of causing distress and allowed the respondents to describe their understanding of their cognitive problems in their own terms. By listening to these descriptions the researcher was able to gain an understanding of the respondent's level of acceptance, insight and knowledge.

WILLINGNESS TO PARTICIPATE

All respondents who consented showed willingness to participate. One refused consent during initial contact. Willingness was shown through a relaxed and interested tone of voice, spontaneity, and verbal comments. One respondent seemed impatient and her answers were cut short and to the point. It is difficult to know what the reasons for this were. Perhaps a face-to-face interview would have provided a different experience and understanding of the situation. The researcher shared this concern with the respondent:

Researcher: I appreciate you giving me some of your time here. We are about halfway through the interview. I can't see you but sense that you might not want to continue? It is OK to stop. I just want to check this out with you.

Respondent: Well I don't mind continuing but I do want to get it over as I have other things I want to do today.

Some respondents did sound a little reluctant or threatened by the research process but when this was shared sensitively, the researcher gathered a clearer understanding of the person and their difficulties. The respondent on the other hand learned that the researcher was not there to judge or force participation.

One male respondent was assertive and questioned the purpose of the interview. The researcher wondered if such assertion was an attempt to cover up anxiety, or a genuine interest in the research process. The researcher answered the respondent's criticisms fully, honestly and non-defensively. Once such issues had been addressed, the researcher checked with the respondent if he wanted to continue with the interview. This was done in a friendly and non-judgemental way. Interestingly the respondent stated:

Respondent: Of course. No one has twisted my arm to participate. (and laughed)

OPENNESS AND CONFIDENTIALITY

Openness is an implicit aim within qualitative research. Encouraging openness requires a degree of trust that must be nurtured during the interview. Achieving such frankness is a challenge to any researcher but is more complex when working with people with dementia, who can experience feelings of suspicion. Such difficulties were modest during this study. Any reluctance or changes in capacity to be open were respected. Rosenfield (1997) suggests that the telephone is 'an excellent medium for enabling the client to feel safe enough to reveal something without feeling too exposed or vulnerable' (p.26).

Computers have also been reported as a medium for interviews (Peiris *et al.* 1995; Williams *et al.* date unknown). Some interviewees were reported to find it easier to reveal sensitive information to a computer than a human interviewer. Williams *et al.* identify the pleasant, non-judgemental and unemotional contact as unique components to the computer assisted interview.

An environment that promotes trust and openness can be created over the telephone by:

> emphasising the confidentiality of the interview and discussing this
>
> clarifying any privacy issues
>
> being skilful, including sensitivity, empathy, warmth, honesty, respectfulness, and a genuine regard for the respondent

compensating for the lack of visual contact through exaggerated verbal gesturing and explicit explanations that can help both parties form a mental picture of each other.

The confidentiality of the interview was explained. The researcher described his/her own working area emphasising privacy, the coding system, note taking and security. The researcher also had to ascertain the privacy of the respondent as this could not be observed. Sometimes the carer was the first point of contact for the researcher. In these cases the researcher would spend some time explaining the project both to the carer and to the respondent. Through social conversation the researcher could check where the respondent would be sitting during the conversation and where the carer would be. Most times carers welcomed the intrusion as they were able to get on with some household duties and left the respondent and researcher to talk. Sometimes the respondent would ask for support from the carer and negotiated their own boundaries of confidentiality. This was managed by either speaking to the carer at various points during the interview, the respondent calling to the carer for help with their memory during the interview, a three-way conversation using a telephone extension line, or speaking to the carer at the end of the interview. Although inclusion of the carer was generally triggered by the respondent, the type of involvement still had to be handled sensitively. All carers were conscious that, and seemed pleased that, the respondent had been invited to participate and did not attempt to take over the conversation. Involvement of carers was mainly for the purpose of clarifying points that the respondent had had difficulty remembering or expressing, or providing additional information.

The following example illustrates issues about openness and confidentiality. It is unknown whether such frankness would have been achieved during a face-to-face interview.

John was extremely easy to converse with. He was not hesitant and had a good grasp of language, answering spontaneously. He spoke about his concerns about having to pay for medication once the 'trial' period was over. He also discussed his financial situation and expressed worries about his rights and paying for care. His wife, who was also in the room (this had been agreed previously), came to the phone during the financial part of the conversation. It became a three-way phone call at this point. The researcher detected some change in their degree of openness. The researcher refocused on the confidentiality of the interview and wondered if they had any doubts as to whether their responses might jeopardise them in some way. Some relief was detected when this became the focus. The conversation was summarised with their help – it captured their confusion about their financial rights but did not detail their finances. They welcomed this 'ownership' and were reassured.

PERSONAL VALUES

Personal values were something that all respondents spoke about with the researcher. Such values were expressed in terms of daily activities and social networks. Discussing such values was a way of expressing identity and was crucial to the aims of the study, which were to understand the needs of people with dementia within a legal context. Expressing personal values helped the researcher to create a mental picture of the respondent that might have been more evident face to face (such as photographs displayed in the living area). Here are three short quotes from respondents indicating how they value autonomy and familial attachment respectively:

> Living on your own – you are more dependent on others. I don't want everyone knowing my affairs.

> The only help I needed was to do with collecting my pension and sorting out my bills. I would approach the nurse – I don't want my relatives to know – they might make a meal of it. It can be very depressing this Alzheimer's stuff.

> I have my family and grandchildren around me. I don't have to think of the future – we all have to go sometime.

Silences

Understanding the reason for silences without being able to see the person has some drawbacks. It is difficult to ascertain if the person is distracted or appears comfortable with the silence, as there is no visual guide. The respondent might be using the silence constructively. The researcher noted that her own tolerance for silences seemed less than during previous face-to-face interviews. Such tendencies are noted by Rosenfield, who suggests that it is more appropriate to break silences at the beginning of relationships. She goes on to sympathise with the dilemmas that occur during silences and suggests that immediate conversation prior to the silence might help to shed light on what is happening during a silence over the telephone.

For people with dementia there is the added difficulty that a silence might be related to difficulties in memory recall. The researcher was sensitive to this specific need and tended to help people through silences, particularly if the person had just indicated that he/she could not remember something. Sometimes the researcher would check out whether the person just needed time to think or needed a prompt.

Creating a mental picture

Both respondent and interviewer created a mental picture of each other. Opportunities to share 'visual' information were used to aid this picture. For example, when a respondent was asked his/her age, some replied with an additional, 'I bet you are just a young thing'. This allowed the researcher to share similar information that would have been more evident from a face-to-face meeting. Other visual sharing opportunities were available at the beginning of the interview when the interviewer checked for comfort and privacy. The researcher informed the respondents about the geographical distance of the call and also the physical environment of the researcher. This provided the respondent with a mental picture, and some informal, peripheral information about the researcher. Geography proved a useful focus and helped to bond the relationship, sharing knowledge of each other's town. This often relaxed respondents quickly and triggered memories of former family holidays. One respondent found this very useful to prompt his memory about his previous employment. This had been difficult for him until the conversation became more social and he started to talk about his days as a photographer in the researcher's locale.

The amount of personal information that should be offered during an interview needs to be balanced. The researcher had to try and compensate for the lack of visual communication. The respondent needed help in creating a mental picture of the researcher in order to make his or her own judgements, which would have been more readily made during a face-to-face interview. Hence, opportunities to share a little of the researcher's own personal profile were sometimes considered appropriate during interviews.

Impact of interview and saying goodbye

Concerns were expressed during ethical clearance about the impact the interview might have on the emotional state of the respondent. The content of the interview was sensitive and potentially emotive. Telephone interviews cannot allow for physical closeness or comfort. Such concerns required careful consideration. Was the telephone a more dangerous medium than a face-to-face interview?

Most interviews appeared to have a positive impact on the respondent. Emotions and changes in emotions were acknowledged. Friendships were formed and several respondents stated that they felt better and/or better informed for speaking with the researcher. The researcher provided telephone helplines, addresses and leaflets where appropriate. Shifts in respondents' thinking did occur:

Respondent: I only see legal advice as being about benefits, wheelchairs – no big issues that I can see…although you have made me think there is more to it, there is more to it than finances – I had not thought about the care side of it in that way.

A crucial safety strategy throughout this project was accessing respondents through CPNs. The advantages of working with CPNs have already been noted and an additional advantage was the support and continuation of support provided by the CPN once the interview was complete. CPNs and respondents were able to discuss the experience of being involved in the research process.

Concern had been expressed by ethical committee members and CPNs about how to say goodbye. If someone was upset, there was a fear that this would be unknown to the researcher and the person would be left afterwards without any support. When the interview was over, the researcher let the respondent know this. Any unfinished business such as the need for further information was dealt with. The researcher also offered feedback to the respondents, particularly those who had voiced concern about their ability to participate:

Researcher: Thank you. I remember you saying at the beginning that you felt you wouldn't have anything to say. You have been most helpful participating in this study and answering my questions. Would you like to ask me anything else?

The researcher proceeded to encourage some social conversation and helped the respondent to focus on their day again. Some respondents had a family member there to support them at the end of the interview. Others lived on their own. The researcher had the option of alerting the CPN to any specific concerns with regard to the respondent. This had to be done without breaking confidentiality. If such liasing was necessary, the researcher would let the CPN know that the respondent had completed the interview and that he/she 'might want to discuss some of this with you'. There was the occasional doubt about a respondent's welfare, just through getting to know the respondent during the telephone call. The calls were not the trigger to these concerns. Such concerns would probably have existed when saying goodbye to the person face to face. Many respondents offered feedback to the researcher:

Respondent: It has been lovely... It is no problem.

Researcher: Do you use the phone much?

Respondent: Just to phone my nephew E in N. I like speaking on the phone.

Conclusions

The telephone as a medium for interviewing people with dementia is effective and potentially empowering. For the researcher it has the advantage of being economical and flexible. For the respondent it offers anonymity, flexibility, control, privacy and accessibility, and is familiar. Limitations to relying on the spoken word alone can be overcome. The skills of the interviewer, the style and flexibility of the interview, and the structure offered can compensate for the lack of visual communication. Difficulties experienced during interviews were not directly related to the telephone as a medium. Most difficulties were related more to cognition and/or more generally to a diversity of barriers that are brought to any interview experience.

However, when working with a potentially vulnerable group of people such as those with dementia, there is a need to detail carefully the protocol for accessing respondents, establishing consent and developing the interview process. Ethical principles must underpin such protocols. Barriers to inclusion have been raised throughout this study and detailed within this chapter, including professional accountability, discrimination and paternalism. All those involved were interested in protecting the person from harm. Identifying CPNs as a safe and professional route to accessing and assessing people with dementia who could use the telephone was crucial to this study. The style of interview developed through the pilot phase was based upon the perspective that social reality is constructed from 'within', respecting the subjective experiences of the person (Cohen and Manion 1989). Thus the aim of the interview was to develop a discourse between the respondent and interviewer that promotes a regard for the social and personal context of the respondent. It was also chosen as a more human experience than standard interview approaches to enable people with cognitive difficulties to engage in the process. Respondents reported positive feelings about telephone interviews and indicated feelings of enjoyment, surprise, increased knowledge and a sense of achievement. One respondent offered the following assessment of their experience of taking part in the study:

> I had no difficulties with the phone call and we got on fine. I quite enjoyed the conversation and it was very helpful. It did me a lot of good and I was quite happy when I came off the phone. My memory can be quite bad and I was pleased to get through the interview without forgetting what I was talking about halfway through. It was a cheery call.

Acknowledgements

Appreciation and thanks to all respondents and carers, to Alzheimer Scotland Action on Dementia (especially Highland) staff, University of Stirling Highland Campus staff and to all the CPNs and managers who supported this study. Without their interest and professionalism people with dementia would never have had the opportunity to participate. A special thank you to Elinor Moore and Anne McKinlay.

Notes

1   The Act sets out to 'empower adults with incapacity, respecting their rights and acknowledging that many have been capable of managing their own affairs in the past and some will be able to do so again in the future' (Adults with Incapacity (Scotland) Bill, Policy Memorandum 1999, p.18).

2   The Centre for Social Research on Dementia at the University of Stirling was commisioned by the Scottish Executive's Central Research Unit.

References

Adults with Incapacity (Scotland) Bill (1999) Policy Memorandum. Edinburgh: The Stationery Office.

Adults with Incapacity Act (2000) Scottish Executive (Scotland) http://www.scottish.parliament-uk/parl_bus/b5as1.pdf

Alzheimer Scotland Action on Dementia (2000) *Planning Signposts for Dementia Care Services.* Alzheimer Scotland Action on Dementia: Edinburgh.

Aneshensel, C., Frerichs, R. R., Clark, V. A. and Yokopenic, P. A. (1982) 'Measuring depression in the community: A comparison of telephone and personal interviews.' *Public Opinion Quarterly 46*, 110–121.

Barak, Y., Macdonald, A. M. and Levy, R. (1998) 'Surveying elderly in the community for Alzheimer's disease.' *Ageing and Mental Health 2*, 2, 87–88.

Bjorn *et al.* (1999) 'Can the written information to research subjects be improved? An empirical study.' *Journal of Medical Ethics 25*, 263–267.

Brandt, J., Spencer, M. and Folstein, M. (1988) 'The telephone interview for cognitive status.' *Neuropsychiatry, Neuropsychology, and Behavioural Neurology 1*, 2, 111–117.

Cohen and Manion (1989) (eds) *Research Methods in Education*, 3rd Edition. London: Routledge

Cotrell, V. and Schulz, R. (1993) 'The perspective of the person with Alzheimer's Disease: A neglected dimension of dementia research.' *Gerontologist 33*, 205–211.

Davis, L. L. (1998) 'Telephone based interventions with family caregivers: A feasibility study.' *Journal of Family Nursing 4*, 3, 255–270.

Department of Health (England and Wales) (1997) *The New NHS: Modern and Dependable.* White Paper. London: HMSO.

Goldsmith, M. (1996) *Hearing the Voice of People with Dementia.* London: Jessica Kingsley Publishers.

Hanson, E., Tetley, J. and Shewan, J. (2000) 'Supporting family carers using interactive multimedia.' *British Journal of Nursing 9*, 11.

Kalisch, B. (1973) 'What is Empathy?' *American Journal of Nursing 73*, 1548–1552.

Keady, J., Gilliard, J., Evers, C. and Milton, S. (1999) 'The DIAL-log study 1: Profiling the experience of people with dementia.' *British Journal of Nursing 8*, 6, 387–393.

Kitwood, T. and Bredin, K. (1992) 'Towards a theory of dementia care: Personhood and well-being.' *Ageing and Society 12*, 269–287.

La Monica, E. (1981) 'Construct validity of an empathy instrument.' *Research in Nursing and Health 4*, 389–400.

Mason, A. (1990) *A study of the relationship between student nurses' and role models' empathy scales.* Unpublished Master of Education degree, Aberdeen.

Mason, A. and Wilkinson, H. (2001) *People with dementia who are users and non-users of the legal system in Scotland: A feasibility study.* Final Report to the Scottish Executive. Stirling: CSRD.

McLaren, P. (1992) 'Psychotherapy by telephone: Experience of patient and therapist.' *Journal of Mental Health 1*, 311–313.

Mishler, E. G. (1986) *Research Interviewing: Context and Narrative.* Cambridge MA: Harvard University Press.

National Health Service and Community Care Act (1990). http://www.hmso.gov.uk/acts/summary/01990019.htm

Patients Charter – A Charter for Health (1998) http://www.cabinet-office.gov.uk/servicefirst/1998/list/scopat.htm

Peiris, D., Alm, N. and Gregor, P. (1995) 'Computer Interviews: An Initial Investigation using Free Text Responses'. In M. Kirby, A. Dix and J. Finlay (eds) *People and Computers X.* Cambridge: Cambridge University Press.

Polit, D. and Hungler, B. (1999) *Nursing Research. Principles and methods.* Sixth edition. Philadelphia: Lippincott.

Pratt, R. and Wilkinson, H. (2000) *No diagnosis has to be your whole life: The effect of being told the diagnosis of dementia from the perspective of the person with dementia.* Final Report to the Mental Health Foundation. Stirling: Centre for Social Research on Dementia.

Priestley, M. (1999) *Disability Politics and Community Care.* London: Jessica Kingsley Publishers.

Revicki, D. A., Tohen, M., Gyulai, L., Thompson, C., Pike, S., Davis-Vogel, A. and Zarate, C. (1997) 'Telephone versus in-person clinical and health status assessment interview in patients with bipolar disorder.' *Harvard Review of Psychiatry 5*, 2, 75–81.

Reynolds, W. (1986) *A Study of Empathy in Student Nurses.* Unpublished Master of Philosophy Degree. Inverness.

Rosenfield, R. (1997) *Counselling by telephone.* London: SAGE Publications.

Slutske, W. S., True, W. R., Scherrer, J. F., Goldberg, J., Bucholz, K. K., Heath, A. C., Henderson, W. G., Eisen, S. A., Lyons, M. J. and Tsaung, M. T. (1998) 'Long term reliability and validity of alcoholism diagnoses and symptoms in a large national telephone interview survey.' *Alcoholism Clinical and Experimental Research 22*, 3, 553–558.

Telephone Helplines Association (1993) *Guidelines for Good Practice in Telephone Work.* London: Telephone Helplines Group/Association.

Williams, B., Peiris, D., Gregor, P., Alm, N., Cumming, S., Flockhart, G. and Groundwater, M. (date unknown) *Computer-based interventions for assisting people who have suffered disabling trauma.* Department of Social Work and Department of Applied Computing: University of Dundee.

Chapter 12

Using video observation to include the experiences of people with dementia in research

Ailsa Cook

Introduction

The recent social policy focus on providing people with dementia with good quality of care has resulted in a drive to find ways to include their experiences in research. These moves have led to a body of researchers experienced in including the perspectives of people with mild dementia in their research (see Allan 2000; Pratt and Wilkinson 2000). To date, however, the experiences of people with moderate and advanced dementia have largely been excluded from research, as it is not known how to facilitate interaction with this group of people with often profoundly impaired communicative abilities.

Much of the research that has sought a window into the lives of people with more advanced dementia has examined their behaviour using systematic observation measures (e.g. Bredin *et al.* 1995; Van Haitsma *et al.* 1997; Ward *et al.* 1992). One of the most widely used of these measures is Dementia Care Mapping (DCM), where the behaviours of people with dementia are coded by an observer into predefined categories, to give a picture of their quality of experience in care (Bredin and Kitwood 1995). This and other systematic observation measures, such as Bowie and Mountain (1993), are limited in that they can only capture aspects of a person's experience as they fall into the predefined categories of behaviour. This research, therefore, cannot offer radically new understandings of the experience of dementia, but merely modify the view of dementia reflected in the researcher's choice of which categories of behaviour to observe.

The reliance on these systematic observation measures has arguably helped to perpetuate a medicalised view of the lives of people with dementia as recipients of care and interaction, be it good or bad. These preconceptions are being challenged by the participation of people with early dementia in the research process and its dissemination (see chapters in this book by Robinson and McKillop). There is, however, an urgent need to find ways to include the experiences of people with dementia in research who are unable to articulate their perspective themselves. This will enable the development of a more realistic and useful model of the experience of dementia with which to inform social care policy and practice.

This chapter describes a research project that used video to include the experiences of people with dementia in research. Specifically the project sought to examine the non-verbal communicative experiences of attendees at a dementia-specific day care centre with varying degrees of cognitive impairment, from mild to fairly advanced. Two researchers observed naturally occurring interactions in the setting using both pen and paper and a video camera to record the observations. Review of the literature on video observation and dementia revealed that it has been used mostly by Scandinavian researchers to examine several aspects of dementia. These include: facial expression (Asplund, Jansson and Norberg 1995; Jannson *et al.* 1992); problems with feeding (Athlin *et al.* 1990; Philips and Van Ort 1993); differential response to stimuli (Norberg, Melin and Asplund 1986); the effectiveness of staff training (Kilhgren *et al.* 1996); and carers strategies for understanding people with dementia (Haggstrom, Jansson and Norberg 1998). Video has been shown to be useful for examining aspects of interaction with people with dementia, and for helping carers reflect on their care. These studies have not, however, used video to explore the experiences of people with dementia other than as they relate to their carers. In addition, none of the studies used video to include the participants with dementia in the research process.

The use of the video-recorder in this study was found to enable the inclusion of the participant with dementia's experiences in the research in two ways. Naturally occurring interactions were video-recorded, providing a detailed and permanent record of the participants' experiences as reflected by their behaviours. These video-recorded observations were not limited by any predefined categories and were analysed qualitatively allowing understandings of the communicative experience to come from the data. Second, the use of video enabled the participants with dementia to be involved in the process of data collection and analysis. The use of a small, light video camera encouraged participants to be involved in the process of filming, and showing the participants the video recordings enabled their interpretations of the behaviours recorded to be included in the research.

This chapter will describe the process of video-recording interactions, including negotiating access to do the research; gaining consent from the participants to be recorded; using the camera; transcribing and analysing the data gathered; and using the videos to elicit interpretations of the interactions from the participants. Problems faced when gathering the data will be discussed. Ethical issues related to capturing and storing the image of someone with dementia will be discussed, in particular as they relate to dissemination of research.

Starting out, negotiating access and gaining consent to do research using video

Before research examining the experiences of people with dementia can be carried out, access must be negotiated with several gatekeepers. Using video to record the daily life in a service setting for older people with dementia is a potentially sensitive enterprise, and it is important to anticipate concerns that gatekeepers may have when negotiating access. The process of negotiating access in this study involved two sets of gatekeepers, the service manager and the social work department, both of whom had similar concerns. These included: the potential intrusiveness of the camera in the setting; how consent would be obtained for the residents with dementia; the extent of staff involvement in the study; that the participants, anonymity would be preserved; and what would happen to the tapes after the research. In addition the service manager was insistent that the relatives be informed of the research, which she said was vital to maintain their continuing cooperation and trust in the service. The social work department also considered how useful the research might be to their work and were keen that the research findings be disseminated to them, including feedback on the success of the consent protocol and other arising ethical issues to be considered when reviewing future research proposals.

After access had been negotiated with the service manager and social work department, a meeting was held with the staff in the service to explain the study and find out if they were willing for it to go ahead in their service. Although it would have been hard for the staff to reject the project altogether, given that they knew it had the support of their manager, this meeting did enable them to highlight concerns they had about the project. In particular, the staff were keen to know what would happen with the videotapes after the study and who would get to see them. They also wanted to know if the project would interfere with their work in any way. Finally several of the staff said that their performance on camera may not reflect the way they normally worked and worried that they would be unable to relax whilst the camera was on.

It is notable that the service users with dementia had no say in whether the project was allowed to go ahead in the service. Instead they were given the option to consent or otherwise to take part in the study, once the approval of the other parties had been given. In this way, the negotiation of access process denied them the chance to say whether they wanted the research project in their service and so actively disempowered them. This situation arose because the researcher could not have access to the attendees to ask them if they were willing for the research to go ahead until access had been agreed with the other gatekeepers.

Having negotiated access with the gatekeepers to carry out the research in the project, individual consent was sought for the attendees in the day centre. In the first instance the researchers approached the attendees formally to tell them about the study and asked if they would be willing to take part. An information sheet was prepared for the participants to keep and the video camera was brought along so the participants could look at it, use it and get a feel for what being recorded might be like. Written consent was not sought from the participants as it was felt unfair to encourage someone with a memory problem to sign a form committing to something that they may forget the details of in time.

The formal consent process was of mixed success: although two of the participants were able to give informed consent to participate in the study, the majority of the participants gave what I have termed 'uninformed consent'. They understood that they had been asked to be involved in a research project and they agreed to take part, without taking the time to understand what this would involve. One participant summed up the response of this group when she said, 'whatever I can do to help, dear'. The mixed success of this approach to gaining consent prompted the researchers also to seek the consent of the participants informally during the field-work process. This was done by reminding the attendees that they were part of a study when appropriate opportunities arose; involving them in watching each other's communication, so they might get a feel for what the study was about; and encouraging them to handle and record with the video camera. Careful attention was paid to both verbal and non-verbal behaviour for indications of the participants' willingness to be involved.

The use of both formal and informal methods enabled the researchers to be reasonably confident that the participants were consenting to take part. This confidence was reinforced by the willingness of participants to indicate when they did not want to talk to the researchers or be recorded. This was done by either getting up and leaving the interaction, or by saying that they wanted to stop the recording when asked. The use of a video camera in the study, however, meant that written consent for participation in the study was also sought from the relatives of those with dementia, even when the attendees themselves had clearly indicated their willingness to participate. Gaining the consent of the participants with dementia alone was not satisfactory in this instance, as the video recordings will be kept for three years (the duration of the project). Therefore, it was essential that someone who would be able to remember that the video existed for at least that period of time was involved in giving consent. To avoid further disempowering the participants with dementia, relatives were only approached for consent after the participant with dementia had indicated that they were willing to take part.

Written informed consent was obtained from the staff members of the service. They were given an information sheet to keep and were reassured that they could decide not to be video-recorded at any time if they chose.

Recording the interactions

Before video-recording interactions, the researchers spent time in the service, joining in the activities and making pen-and-paper observations about the communication occurring in the day centre. Informal consent was regularly negotiated during this time and the participants were involved in observing each other. In this way they began to develop an understanding of the study and the researchers' role in the day centre. This period spent observing and chatting to the participants with dementia and the staff proved essential to the smooth introduction of the video camera to the day centre.

Video recordings were then taken of naturally occurring situations. The researchers based their decision as to which interactions to record on convenience and interest. Before recording an interaction, the researchers would approach the group and explain that they wished to record the activity. The camera was passed round so that the participants with dementia could record each other and get a feel for what being part of the project was like. The participants were told that if they chose, they could watch the video the following week. They were also reassured that the video camera could be turned off at any time if they wanted. Having obtained the consent of all the participants, both those with dementia and the staff, one of the researchers joined in the group and took some notes whilst the other video-recorded the action.

The room that the activities were conducted in limited the filming to a degree. The room was quite cramped, and therefore not all of a group could be recorded at once. This problem was overcome by moving with the video camera to record different groups of individuals in turn. Ideally the camera should be positioned with natural light behind it, about two metres from the subject of the picture; however, the quality of the digital handheld camera meant that good pictures were obtained from all angles and distances. The recordings focused primarily on the person at the centre of the interaction at the time, and included as many as possible of the other participants. The camera had a good quality zoom, so close-up shots of participants' facial expressions could be taken as needed without placing the camera near their faces.

During the video recordings the participants were reminded of the presence of the camera and asked if they were willing for recording to continue. Often the participants had forgotten about the camera, and always said that they were happy for it to be there. Although they were not bothered by the camera, the participants with dementia did signal when they wanted the interaction that was being recorded to end, either by saying so, when asked, or by getting up and leaving. The staff, however, did seem more conscious of the presence of the camera, and were recorded glancing at the camera from time to time, which is something that the participants with dementia never did.

Reviewing interactions with the participants

The participants with and without dementia were asked after the recordings if they would like to watch the video. This was done on a different day, as the film had to be copied onto standard videotape to be played through the day centre's video player. Access to a more modern television in the setting would have enabled the videos to be shown immediately after the recording as the camera could have been plugged into the back of the television. The videos were only shown to the people who participated in the recording, if everyone in the recording agreed that they were willing for the videos to be shown. In one case a participant clearly stated, when asked, that he did not want to see the film, but said that he was happy for the staff member recorded and the researcher to watch it together.

Reviewing the videos enabled the participants with dementia to provide interpretations of specific interactions and behaviours recorded on camera. In one instance, four participants with dementia and two staff were video-recorded playing a board game. When asked, all participants said they would like to watch the video the following week. Three of the four participants with dementia could identify themselves and each other, however the fourth participant identified everyone else, but did not identify herself. She did however mimic her gestures on the screen, and no one else's, suggesting that she knew at least at some level that this was her. When asked, the attendees identified behaviours such as whispering in the ear to another, and interpreted this as cheating at the game. The participant who didn't acknowledge her presence on the screen still offered interpretations of her behaviour. She interpreted her gesture of sitting with her hands covering her face when not able to answer a question as 'hiding'. Similarly one participant identified another's elaborate hand movements when rolling the dice as 'his banter'. These interpretations were useful as they confirmed the researchers' interpretations and showed that the participants could pick up on subtle social cues in the interaction, even if they couldn't remember the interaction happening, and couldn't identify themselves.

Showing the videos to the staff also enabled them to offer their interpretations of the communication observed. When shown the video, they were able to reflect on the interaction in depth, and identified which parts they were pleased with and what they would have done differently a second time. One staff member questioned his use of a book during the interaction and noticed how his physical positioning had been hindering the conversation. He also commented on the success with which he had reinforced some of the participant's non-verbal behaviours and had let her keep talking even though he hadn't fully understood the meaning of what she was saying. These interviews were tape-recorded for later transcription and analysis.

Some of the staff involved in the review process reported that this procedure was beneficial to their practice. Watching the video recordings enabled them to reflect on their behaviour and look at their communication in a different way. During the review process staff reflected on their communication in a critical and positive way and developed more sophisticated understandings of the interaction than they had been operating with during the interaction itself. One of the attendees, however, found the review process unsettling, possibly because she was aware that she was on the television, but had forgotten being filmed and so how she had got there. This unease may have been lessened if the researchers had been clearer when introducing the activity to the attendees.

Transcription and analysis

The transcription and analysis process started by reviewing the videotapes to determine the types of interaction occurring. Excerpts from the video recordings containing notable examples of different types of interaction were then transcribed verbatim. These transcriptions included verbal and non-verbal communication, physical positioning of the participants, and context of the interactions, including what was happening before the video camera was turned on. Three layers of extra information were then added to the transcriptions. First, the researchers' interpretations of the observed behaviours were included; for example that Sidney is playing with the dice to draw attention away from the fact that he doesn't know the answer. Second, the interpretations of the participants were added, in this case that the game with the dice was his 'banter'. Finally the reflections of the interaction partners without dementia prompted by this episode were included.

The process of producing a transcript in this way is very time-consuming, but has the advantage that the experiences of the people with dementia in the frame can be examined in detail. It also allows for the interpretations of the communication of both the participants with and without dementia to be included in the research. This depth of analysis enabled the development of a complex picture of the experience of dementia in this setting. The understandings that emerged following this process included a picture of the participants showing nerves as their turn in the game came, and using primarily humour to hide the fact that they didn't know the answers. Less impaired participants were observed to add to the humour by colluding with them and telling them the answers. Non-verbal gestures were used to both answer questions, such as miming of swimming, and to distract people's attention from their failure to answer the questions. Staff and participants with dementia used non-verbal behaviours to support and reassure each other as they struggled to find the answers.

One problem faced in the analysis was that their presence at and partic-ipation in the interaction as it was being filmed influenced the researchers' interpretations of the interaction. When the videos were shown to members of the research team who were not involved in the fieldwork they interpreted certain aspects of the interaction differently to the researchers and the participants who had been present. This discrepancy occurred for two key reasons. First, the video recording could not include all the responses of everyone involved in the interaction all the time. This infor-mation was added later to the transcriptions, but at a much lesser depth than would have been obtained had these responses been recorded. Possibly more importantly, however, the members of the research team not involved in the fieldwork were not aware of the wider context in which the interactions occurred. They watched the video with no knowledge of the interpersonal dynamics of the setting, or the kinds of jokes that went on. Knowledge of this context obviously strongly coloured the interpretations of the researchers who had been in the fields of interaction.

Ethical issues related to using video in research

Aside from the problem of gaining the participants' consent, there are a number of ethical issues to be considered when using video in research. Using video observation to record people's experiences places the research participant in a vulnerable position, as they give the researcher a resource that could be used to their disadvantage. This potential for harm, inten-tional or inadvertent, is greater for those who are disempowered or face social exclusion, as many people with dementia and the staff who work with them do. It was clear from this research that many of the participants had not considered the damaging ways in which the video recordings could be used and trusted the researchers to act in their best interests. Careful consideration of these issues has led to the identification of three key ways in which the researcher may wittingly or unwittingly place his/her participants in a compromising position or add to their exclusion and disempowerment.

During the research process, there is a danger that the video may be used in a way that objectifies the research participants or their experiences, and emphasises their 'otherness', thereby adding to their exclusion and disadvantage (Fine 1994). Previous research using video to investigate aspects of dementia has been guilty of this, by using the camera to examine the experiences of the 'subjects' as if they were in a goldfish bowl. Smith (1995), for example, video-recorded people with dementia and 'normal controls' watching video clips and analysed the recordings using a coding schedule to see if people with dementia (viewed as a homogenous, diagnostic group) responded to others' emotion with facial expression. In this way the research objectified the individuals involved as members of a diagnostic category with a specific communicative dysfunction. Fine (1994) stresses how this type of research objectifies the participants and serves to add to the exclusion that disadvantaged groups face. Instead, she calls for researchers to include the participants' voices in research and emphasise the heterogeneity of their experiences. Therefore it is essential, if the research is to facilitate inclusion, that the participants' perspectives are ascertained wherever possible.

This research sought to include the perspectives of the participants by showing them the videos and asking them to offer interpretations of the interactions recorded. It is important, however, that the video recordings of the participants with and without dementia are not shown to families or other people in that setting, unless they too were involved in the interaction. Participants with dementia in our recordings were observed to use humour and gestures in ways that might appear to be childlike or crude when taken out of context, and staff were seen to encourage these forms of expression. Showing these recordings to others involved in the setting, but not that particular interaction, leaves both the staff and attendees open to judgement and may prevent the participants from continuing to express themselves in ways which may be unacceptable in other settings. In particular, families may be unwilling to accept the ways in which their relative behaves when in a day-centre setting with others of their own age as opposed to in the family home.

Given the potentially stigmatising nature of a diagnosis of dementia, it is equally important that the images of people with dementia are not shown to people in the wider community, unless permission is expressly given from the people with dementia themselves. The powerful visual images captured on camera could be used to enhance the dissemination of the research, for example in conference presentations or training videos; however, this both identifies who the research participants are and that they have dementia. This means that it is no longer within the person with dementia's control who does and does not know their diagnosis. Furthermore, that person is inherently linked to any interpretation that the researcher puts on the data, regardless of whether he/she agrees with it or not. Putting images of people with dementia on the internet is potentially even more damaging, as it not only increases the numbers of people who may identify that individual as having dementia but unless extreme care is taken, others may download the image and use it in ways neither the researcher nor the participant can control.

The ethical issues surrounding the dissemination of research have led the research team to consider alternative methods for representing the interactions recorded in the project, so that the findings may be presented visually without compromising the anonymity of the participants. Pilot work is in progress at the University of Stirling in conjunction with the Royal Scottish Academy of Music and Drama to determine the possibility of using actors to represent the observed interactions. Older actors will be shown excerpts of video and asked to reproduce the interactions seen. This is a costly and time-consuming process, which includes writing storyboards, hiring a director, actors and film crew, organising costumes and make up, editing the films and transferring the material onto CD-ROM and video. Once completed, it is hoped that the films may be used to disseminate the findings visually in online papers, conference presentations and training materials.

Conclusions

Video observation can be used to include the experiences of people with moderate and advanced dementia in research. Using video observation not only made it possible to document and analyse in depth the experiences of people with dementia, it also facilitated their participation in the research process. Furthermore, review and analysis of the video recordings enabled the researchers and participants to reach a deeper understanding of the interactions than would have been obtained through participation in the interactions alone.

Carrying out research using video is a time-consuming enterprise. The potential vulnerability of the participants whose images are recorded on video demands that special care be taken when negotiating access and consent to do the research. Gatekeepers and research participants must be made aware of the ethical issues particular to using video in research and be assured that appropriate protocols are in place, especially for preserving the anonymity of the participants. Spending time in the setting before starting to record the interactions is also important so that the participants feel comfortable enough with the research to take some control of it. This is essential to ensure that the video is used to include and empower the participants as opposed to objectifying their experiences. Finally, transcription and analysis is a lengthy process, made longer by the inclusion of the participants' perspectives on the interactions.

Used carefully, video observation is a powerful research tool, which can add to our understandings of the experience of dementia and make the inclusion of people with dementia in research a reality. Consideration of the ethical issues particular to using video in research is essential, however, to ensure that being video-recorded is a positive experience for all involved.

Acknowledgments

I would like to acknowledge the collaboration of Gill Hubbard, who was involved in the design, data collection and analysis of the project described in this chapter. I would also like to acknowledge the supervision I have received from Heather Wilkinson, Gwyneth Doherty-Sneddon and Susan Tester.

References

Allan, K. (2000) *Hearing the views of people with dementia about the services they receive.* Paper given to the Journal of Dementia Care Conference, 6 April, Edinburgh.

Asplund, K., Jansson, L. and Norberg. A. (1995) 'Facial expressions of patients with dementia: A comparison of two methods of interpretation.' *International Psychogeriatrics 7*, 4, 527–534.

Athlin, E., Norberg, A., Asplund, K. and Jansson, L. (1990) 'Feeding problems in severely demented patients seen from task and relationship aspects.' *Scandinavian Journal of Caring Sciences 3*, 3, 113–121.

Bowie, P. and Mountain, G. (1993). 'Using direct observation to record the behaviour of long-stay patients with dementia.' *International Journal of Geriatric Psychiatry 8*, 12, 857–864.

Bredin, K., Kitwood, T. and Wattis, J. (1995) 'Decline in quality of life for patients with severe dementia following a ward merger.' *International Journal of Geriatric Psychiatry 10*, 967–973.

Fine, M. (1994) 'Working with Hyphens: Reinventing self and other in qualitative research.' In N. K. Denzin and Y. S. Lincoln (eds) *Handbook of Qualitative Research.* Thousand Oaks, California: Sage.

Haggstrom, T., Jansson, L. and Norberg, A. (1998). 'Skilled carer's ways of understanding people with Alzheimer's Disease.' *Scholarly Inquiry for Nursing Practice 12*, 3, 239–266.

Jansson *et al.* (1992) 'Interpreting facial expressions in patients in the terminal stages of Alzheimer's Disease.' *Omega 26*, 24, 309–324.

Kihlgren, M., Hallgren, A., Norberg, A. and Karlsson, I. (1996) 'Disclosure of basic strengths and weaknesses in demented patients during morning care.' *International Journal of Ageing and Human Development 43*, 3, 219–233.

Norberg, A., Melin, E. and Asplund, K. (1986) 'Reactions to music, touch and object presentation in the final stage of dementia: An exploratory study.' *International Journal of Nursing Studies 23*, 4, 315–323.

Phillips, L. R. and Van Ort, S. (1993) 'Measurement of mealtime interaction among persons with dementing disorder.' *Journal of Nursing Measurement 1*, 1, 41–55.

Pratt, R. and Wilkinson, H. (2000) *The effect of being told the diagnosis of dementia from the perspective of the person with dementia.* Paper presented at the British Society of Gerontology Annual Conference, Oxford, September.

Smith, M. C. (1995) 'Facial expression in mild dementia of the Alzheimer's type.' *Behavioural Neurology 8*, 149–156.

Van Haitsma, K., Powell, Lawton, M., Kleban, M. H., Klapur, J. and Corn, J. (1997) 'Methodological aspects of the study of streams of behaviour in elders with dementing illness.' *Alzheimer's Disease and Associated Disorders 11*, 4, 228–238.

Ward, T., Murphy, E., Procter, A. and Weinman, J. (1992) 'An observational study of two long-stay psychogeriatric wards.' *International Journal of Geriatric Psychiatry 7*, 211–217.

South Asian people with dementia
Research issues

Alison M. Bowes and Heather Wilkinson

Introduction

For South Asian people, dementia has been characterised as a 'hidden problem' (Brownlie 1991). Dementia is a condition without a name in many South Asian languages, and an experience that is seldom brought into public view. Yet in the coming years, as the UK South Asian population ages, more people will experience dementia, and will have need for understanding of the condition, as well as for support from services for themselves, their families and their carers. Currently, mainstream (i.e. non-minority) services are widely documented as being extremely limited in their ability to respond to South Asian people with dementia (Anderson and Brownlie 1997 give a number of examples). Specialist services are few, and tend to be project-based, time-limited by funding constraints, and to command limited resources.

In this chapter, we explore existing knowledge about South Asian people with dementia, with particular reference to their needs for and use of services. Having established the contributions and limitations of this existing knowledge, we go on to identify the potential for increasing this knowledge base through research, and some of the issues that face researchers doing work in this area. In the process, we draw on our records of research with South Asian older people and with people with dementia, suggesting ways of addressing the many difficult issues which research with South Asian people with dementia presents. Throughout, we discuss issues in relation to wider debates concerning research with vulnerable and marginalised groups. The focus on South Asian people (i.e. those with a heritage in the Indian sub-continent) allows us to explore cultural and linguistic issues in reference to a population which, whilst being diverse in many aspects of language and culture, including religion, also demonstrates some shared issues that reflect minority ethnic status in the UK. These shared issues include exclusion, racism, lack of access to and lack of use of services. Some areas of discussion will be relevant to all those with minority ethnic status; others are specific to the South Asian category or to the various groups within it. The research data discussed were collected in Scotland, but our conclusions can be generalised to other parts of the UK, as we will demonstrate.

Current knowledge: population and incidence

The older South Asian population in the UK is as yet relatively small, as the migrant populations of the 1950s and 1960s are only now entering older age. There are currently very few South Asian people in their eighties and nineties, when the incidence of dementia in the general population reaches its height. But as the South Asian population ages in the coming years, numbers in the older age groups will increase, because each age cohort is progressively larger (cf. Ahmad and Walker 1997; Lindesay *et al.* 1997a).

Yet little is known of the precise dimensions of the potential South Asian population with dementia. There are a number of reasons for this. First, there are weaknesses in the demographic data collected on older South Asian people. Investigations following the 1991 Census identified a 'missing million' people who had not been counted, and there is some evidence to suggest that this group may have included the oldest South Asian people, especially women (Simpson 1996). Thus calculations of the numbers of older people are subject to significant error.

Second, difficulties in calculating numbers of people with dementia are caused by lack of reliable epidemiological data. In the general population, it is known that a significant minority of older people will develop dementia (1.5 per cent at 65, rising to about 33 per cent at 90+ –

Huismann, Raven and Geiger 1998, p.8). Huismann *et al.* (1998, p.14) calculated that about 7 per cent of older people of migrant origin aged 65 and over are likely to develop dementia. They were unable to indicate how these figures might break down further, simply due to lack of data.

Third, the identification of dementia is particularly problematic for South Asian cultures, which do not recognise dementia as a specific condition, but classify it with other mental disorders as 'madness'. Yeo, Gallagher-Thompson and Lieberman (1996) discuss problems of diagnosis in an American multicultural context. They argue that different responses to the experience of dementia by different cultural groups affect whether help, either in the form of diagnosis or of support from services outside the family, is sought.

Fourth, there is some evidence that risk of dementia varies between populations. Larson and Imai (1996) reviewed epidemiological studies that appeared to demonstrate such variation, again in an American context. This variation did not appear to result from problems of diagnosis, which might affect incidence rates. Mungas' (1996) research on Hispanic Americans suggests that they may be more susceptible to vascular dementia, and that this is linked with their tendency towards cardiovascular problems and high incidence of diabetes. British South Asians, who exhibit both these tendencies (Nazroo 1997), may also be at higher risk, though data are insufficiently robust to draw firm conclusions.

Thus, quantitative data on dementia among South Asians in the UK are lacking. There have been some attempts to explore the incidence of dementia qualitatively, in the face of difficulties such as those outlined. For example, Brownfoot (1998) conducted a qualitative study of people with dementia from different minority ethnic groups, including Indians, in Haringey, London. This study demonstrated that people with dementia in minority communities tended to be hidden, that it was essential to work through trusted contacts to identify them and that their needs and preferences remained unknown. This work begins to indicate how South Asian people with dementia might be identified, and also shows many of the difficulties likely to be experienced. In common with other studies (such as Lindesay *et al.* 1997b), this work did not reach the point of getting the views of people with dementia themselves. Success in identifying people with dementia is not always achieved. Boneham *et al.* (1997), for example, using a snowballing technique following up contacts made through GP surgeries aimed to identify a 'total enumeration' of older people from ethnic minorities in Liverpool. This population was then screened to identify people with 'case level' (i.e. requiring intervention) depression or dementia. Only one South Asian person was subsequently identified. Many of the interviews for this study were conducted using interpreters or proxy interviewers. As we will argue below, such an approach is often seen to have serious limitations; Boneham *et al.*'s (1997) study suggests that on many occasions, alternatives may not be feasible.

Others have approached the issue by focusing on service providers (e.g. Anderson and Brownlie 1997; Brownlie 1991; Huismann *et al.* 1998; Patel *et al.* 1998), exploring their experiences of providing services. In general, such studies have found a lack of appropriate services, little use of such services as are available, and a tendency for services to be called in when a crisis occurs, and family carers are unable to cope. Whilst service use prompted by crisis may also occur in the general population, there is good reason to conclude that it is particularly characteristic of South Asians and other minorities, who have been demonstrated to encounter other mental health services in a similar way (Nazroo 1999; Sashidharan and Francis 1993). Such a conclusion emphasises that experiences of dementia among South Asian people in the UK are more common than use of services might suggest. It is reinforced by the much more general lack of use of services for older people, which has been widely demonstrated (e.g. Blakemore and Boneham 1994; Bowes and Dar 2000).

There is no clear evidence that screening instruments used for the general population will prove effective for South Asians. Problems in the cross-cultural application of such instruments are well documented for many disorders (Pilgrim and Rogers 1999), and it is not surprising that these problems are carried over into the dementia field. The only test currently available in South Asian languages is the MMSE,[1] which has been tested in Gujarati by Lindesay *et al.* (1997b), and in other languages, including Urdu/Punjabi, the main languages of South Asians in Scotland, by Rait *et al.* (2000). It has not been subject to full validation – Rait *et al.*'s sample included only 39 Urdu/Pakistani people (p.56). Experience elsewhere, documented by a series of American studies (Baker 1996; Mungas 1996; Taussig and Pontón 1996; Teng 1996), indicates that the development of culturally appropriate instruments, whilst requiring much skilful investigation and testing, is both possible and effective. There is also some evidence that MMSE can be successfully adapted for use with non-literate people (Ganguli *et al*. 1995; Kabir and Herlitz 2000; Tsolaki *et al*. 2000).

As well as being influenced by cultural variation, possible differences of incidence and difficulties of assessment, recognition of dementia among South Asians in the UK is also subject to influence by processes of exclusion. These processes include lack of accessible services, which we discuss further below.

Current knowledge: relevant research

There is a record of research on older South Asian people, on people with mental health problems, and on disability in South Asian communities, which offers insights relevant to work on dementia.

South Asian older people are frequently portrayed by researchers as being especially badly off, experiencing Norman's (1985) 'triple jeopardy' of age discrimination, racism and poverty, and inaccessible services. Butt and Mirza's (1996) review reiterates this perspective, but Blakemore (2000) has recently challenged it, arguing that of all minorities, South Asians are best placed to meet the needs of older people from their communities. He demonstrates that, at face value at least, these communities have a large proportion of young people, forming a large pool of potential family carers. However, this argument underestimates the importance of the relative poverty of people from labour-migrant origins (Butt and Mirza 1996), generally poorer housing conditions, which may exacerbate difficulties related to disability and ill-health (Carlin 1999), and evidence of changing family structures, which may leave older people with diminishing opportunities for potential family care (Ahmad 1996). Furthermore, wider research on carers, including carers in South Asian communities (e.g. Atkin and Rollings 1993; Parker and Lawton 1994; Twigg 1992) has established that carers can experience considerable difficulties in their caring work, and that they need support from outside the family. Recent studies (e.g. Netto 1996, 1997) and policy and practice guidance (e.g. Commission for Racial Equality 1997; Department of Health SSI 1998) have attempted to challenge the stereotypical view that South Asian families and communities 'look after their own', and to argue that South Asian carers need accessible, culturally appropriate, services.

For South Asian older people who have dementia, it is clear that the difficulties experienced by older people in general will be multiplied. They face at least a 'quadruple jeopardy', with cognitive disability added to Norman's (1985) three factors, listed earlier. In the context of lack of recognition of dementia within South Asian communities, their difficulties are especially severe. Similarly, caring for a person with dementia is, in Parker and Lawton's (1994) terms, an example of the most arduous form of care, involving long hours, great responsibility, likelihood of living in the same house as the person cared for, and performance of more caring tasks. As we noted above, there are indications that the availability of family care in South Asian communities may diminish. One relevant factor here is the gender ratio of older South Asian people, there being more older men than older women, and a significant, though hard to reach, population of older men who never married and live alone. Furthermore, there is some evidence that family structures are changing, and that Indian older people are increasingly likely to be living away from their extended families (Ahmad 1996). This trend is far less significant in Pakistani and Bangladeshi families. But diminishing family care coupled with lack of appropriate services can only increase difficulties.

A wide range of mental health problems in South Asian communities have been the subject of research attention, though dementia has not generally been included. A key problem identified in this literature has been that of diagnosis (discussed above), with standard assessment instruments being especially difficult to use (Nazroo 1999, p.84).

Recent work has started to focus on people's own perceptions and accounts of their mental health and mental distress – Scottish examples include Srivastava and Bowes (1996) and Donaghy (1997). Such work demonstrates that discussion of mental health is possible in research with South Asians. The research has been qualitative, and has explored understandings of mental health and illness, and associated service use. In relation to depression, Donaghy (1997) emphasised the importance of examining experiences of depression in their social context, finding evidence of disappointed aspirations in many of the second generation young women he interviewed. The problems were directly related to ethnicity, but also to the strain of living with the pressures of poverty and racism. Srivastava and Bowes' (1996) work illustrated that older South Asian people experiencing mental distress sought help from their GPs and also from the community-based groups that were providing services designed specifically for South Asian clients. Both these sources of help were seen to be relatively sympathetic.

Disability is a little researched area for UK South Asians, though there is some limited work on people with learning disabilities. Few studies attempt to examine the views of people themselves (Azmi et al. 1996, 1997; Bignall and Butt 2000), whereas the views of carers are more likely to be studied (Butt and Mirza 1996). Some studies have explored the incidence of learning disabilities amongst South Asians, which is disputed. Butt and Mirza (1996) argue that apparently higher rates of learning disabilities may be due to poorer socio-economic conditions, but that many explanations have focused on particular cultural practices such as consanguineous marriage. They therefore alert us to the need to examine both external, environmental factors as well as specific cultural practices when researching disabilities, and reinforce the notion that disabled South Asian people experience multiple burdens. Azmi et al. (1997), who interviewed South Asian adults and adolescents about their service needs and uses, also argue along these lines, identifying a double discrimination of ethnicity and disability.

Butt and Mirza (1996) draw attention to the risks of too strong an emphasis on the negative attitudes in South Asian communities towards learning disabilities. They argue that reports of negative attitudes may reflect stereotypes held by service providers, which are used to explain low take-up of services and excuse failure to offer appropriate services. There is certainly a need for care in the potential uncritical application of general views about South Asian cultures. Recent research at Stirling, which included work with South Asian people with learning disabilities and their families, demonstrated that though there were indeed negative attitudes within the South Asian communities, and that families preferred to keep their experiences private, it was not these attitudes that prevented them from gaining access to services, but lack of information, social isolation and lack of services perceived as accessible (Bowes, Sim and Srivastava 2001).

In the light of this research in other, related areas, it would be a mistake to see South Asian cultures as fixed, and to come to the view that perspectives on dementia cannot change. In the UK context, there has been gradual acceptance of specialist services for older South Asian people, and in Glasgow, for example, day centres are widely used and enjoyed (Bowes and Dar 2000). Blakemore and Boneham's (1994) review demonstrates other developments of this kind, and Blakemore (2000) has recently argued that the experiences of exclusion in South Asian communities are significantly tempered by community resources, including the active voluntary sector, which has developed culturally appropriate services. In terms of mental health issues, there is some evidence that disorders are being increasingly acknowledged, and that the stigma attached to them is decreasing. A good example is that of depression which, whilst still attracting some negative reactions, is much more widely recognised, with people more inclined to seek help (Donaghy 1997). Also relevant are changes in attitudes to caring. More traditionally, care was seen as the sole duty of a person's family. Whilst this remains a strong view, there is some research evidence that family carers want and need support, and will take advantage of it where it is available (Bowes and Dar 2000; Netto 1996, 1997). Changes in family structure and ways of life are also making traditional patterns of caring more difficult to sustain, especially in Indian families, which tend to be smaller than Muslim families from Pakistan and Bangladesh. Changes such as these offer prospects for greater recognition and understanding of dementia, and for people to seek support outside the family. Furthermore, the existence of the Alzheimer's Society of India, and the gradual development of support for people with dementia in the sub-continent (10/66 Dementia Research Group 2000a, 2000b) offers further evidence for the potentiality of change.

Research issues

As our discussion already suggests, a key problem in research with South Asian people with dementia is identifying them. This is an example of a hidden population of extremely vulnerable people. Research on the topic could also be seen as potential cultural interference, involving alterations in perceptions of the condition, and recognition of an otherwise unrecognised problem.

A number of methodological issues arise when research with South Asian people with dementia is contemplated. They include the identification of respondents, issues of language and culture, and consent. We will argue that ways forward lie in collaborative working and a focus on the person with dementia.

Identifying respondents

As a hidden population, South Asian people with dementia present the researcher with all the classic problems of such populations when attempts are made to identify respondents. Dementia may be concealed from outsiders, being a source of stigma and shame. Therefore the establishment of trust is critical, and the use of trusted intermediaries likely to be essential. Such intermediaries may be professionals in health or social work services, who may be supporting South Asian people with dementia. Or they may be trusted members of local communities, such as workers in the voluntary sector. The most likely way to contact respondents is through snowball sampling, and this has indeed been used in earlier studies (e.g. Boneham *et al.* 1997; Brownfoot 1998). Our own work with older South Asian people (Bowes and Dar 1996, 2000) has also used this approach.[2]

In our experience, the use of intermediaries is attractive because it offers a practical way of identifying a population that is otherwise hard to reach. However, it poses a number of problems. First, there are issues of confidentiality. Respondents have sometimes been mistrustful of researchers, questioning them closely about their relationships with the intermediaries, and seeking reassurance that their views will not be passed on. Frequently, reference is made to the closeness of the South Asian communities, and the ability for news to travel fast. Workers in community organisations with which we have worked are seen very much as part of the South Asian communities, and less as detached, objective professionals. Dar, who conducted interviews for the research, also found herself on occasion mistaken for a social worker, a person to whom respondents did not wish to disclose their views.

Second, gatekeepers are in many ways rightly protective of the people with whom they work, who are often particularly vulnerable. They also experience frequent requests for interviews, without necessarily being fully informed about their purpose or their potential results – this experience is at least partly due to the convenience of using gatekeepers to contact samples. Careful negotiation with gatekeepers is therefore likely to be necessary, and access is not assured. In some cases, the concern of gatekeepers extends further. In the voluntary sector in particular, there is competition for contracts and funding (Reid Howie Associates 2001) and, in some cases, clients – for example, recent geographical changes in voluntary sector services for older people in Glasgow have resulted in no provision in one part of the city and extra facilities in another (Bowes *et al.* 2001). This competition can result in gatekeepers developing an almost proprietorial interest in 'their' clients, and becoming less than willing to 'share' them with outsiders. This of course has some implications for the clients, whose autonomy in decisions about participation in research may thus be compromised.

A third issue in identifying respondents is that of diagnosis. We have already discussed difficulties of diagnosing dementia in South Asian people, and suggested that they are less likely to have a diagnosis than are those in the general population (who in any case often fail to be diagnosed for years – Downs 1996). If diagnosis is a criterion for inclusion in a study, the numbers potentially identified will be yet smaller. They may also be people with whom it is more difficult to work, whose dementia is more advanced, to the point at which families have been forced to seek outside help because of some crisis. Our recent discussion with professionals working with South Asian people with dementia has suggested that the use of the term 'memory problems' is helpful in discussing dementia, and that it can be translated into relevant languages. But having 'memory problems' is not equivalent to a diagnosis of dementia, and researchers must face issues of who exactly is to be included in their studies and why. It is worth noting in this connection that the social dimensions of dementia are thrown into particularly sharp relief by these problems, in that the search for understanding, the identification of service need and the development of appropriate services are not wholly determined by or achievable from a starting point of medical diagnosis.

Issues of language and culture

Much of the research we reviewed earlier in the chapter emphasises the importance of language and culture to research on South Asian older people, mental health issues and learning disabilities. For most South Asian older people in the UK, the use of their own language is essential in collecting their views, and researchers require familiarity with South Asian cultures to facilitate effective communication and to make sense of people's comments. It is commonplace in such work to use interviewers who are 'matched' by language and ethnicity, and often also by gender, to respondents. For example, this was done in the major Fourth National Survey of Ethnic Minorities in Britain (Modood *et al.* 1997). This practice is not free of problems, as Rhodes' (1994) arguments suggest. First, a 'matched' interviewer may be perceived as an insider, a member of the local community and hence part of its gossip network. This perception will emphasise the issues of confidentiality we discussed earlier.

Second, shared language and culture are advantageous, but they do not guarantee understanding. An assumption that they do involves a stereotypical view of South Asian cultures as static, homogeneous and undifferentiated. In fact, as we have argued, they are dynamic, heterogeneous and differentiated. Those South Asian people who now have dementia were migrants, with a particular set of experiences that their children will not have. This difference alone profoundly affects people's views of the world, and generational differences can be assumed to exist. Furthermore, socio-economic differentiation within South Asian communities confers different life chances and life experiences. Within each of the commonly used Census categories of Indian, Pakistani and Bangladeshi, there are many different ethnic groups. The basis for deep understanding in an

interview involves the discovery of 'common ground' between interviewer and interviewee, which is not achieved by matching a limited
range of characteristics. It involves highly developed interviewing skills
(Kvale 1996). Shah's (1999) experiences are of some interest here. An
experienced, Gujarati-speaking psycho-geriatrician, he recounts great difficulties interviewing Gujarati older people in their own language, and
attributes these to such issues as the age gap between himself and his
patients, the limitations of Gujarati vocabulary for discussing mental
health issues, the cultural unfamiliarity of some of the medical assessment
techniques he was using, the hospital environment and the tendency for
people's families to take the older person's difficulties as unproblematic,
requiring no help or treatment.

Third, communication with people with dementia is not simply
achieved by sharing their language and culture. Allan (2001) has recently
explored a series of techniques care workers may use to improve communication in their work with people with dementia. Many of these are concerned with gaining a better understanding of the person's views and
feelings, allowing the care worker to respond to people more effectively,
thus improving the quality of care. Researchers can learn from the fund of
practical experience held by those who work with people with dementia
about better ways of communicating with people, and of ascertaining their
views.

Consent

Other chapters in this volume have discussed issues of gaining informed
consent from people with dementia in some detail, and all the issues they
identify also apply in the case of South Asian people. In addition, work
with South Asians perhaps involves further problems. A key example is
that of illiterate respondents, who cannot read information (which, of
course, researchers carefully provide in translated form), and cannot
provide the signed consent requested by many research ethics committees.
These people challenge researchers to rethink their traditional tools for
obtaining informed consent. For example, information about projects can
be supplied on cassette tapes, which can be loaned to potential respon-

dents. Consent to participate might also be recorded, and the respondents asked to give their names. Few social researchers would be satisfied however with a signed consent form, or a cassette recording. The British Sociological Association Code of Ethical Practice presents research consent as requiring continuing negotiation as a project proceeds, and this is widely supported in the research literature. Looked at from this perspective, the illiterate respondent is less of an issue, since, like all respondents, they require continuing negotiation of informed consent.

Ways forward for future research

Research on the general population with dementia (reviewed by Downs and Marshall 1997; Marshall 1999) has demonstrated that specialist services in this area are few; there has been a general lack of audit activity so that little is known about populations with dementia; there is a need for earlier diagnosis of dementia; there are high levels of unmet need for services; and more effective management and coordination of services is necessary. This work suggests that dementia presents particular issues for service provision that are different from, as well as complementary to, those attached to community care and related areas of service.

There is some debate in the literature concerning whether the needs of those from minority ethnic groups are different from those of the general population. Ahmad and Atkin (1996) argue that whilst research on minority and majority groups proceeds along rather different lines, this debate is unlikely to be resolved. Bowes and MacDonald (2000) compare findings on majority and minority ethnic older people, concluding that there were both similarities between and variations within each group, and suggesting that the development of person-centred (rather than culturally targeted) services is appropriate for both. It is essential that comparisons are maintained between the general population and minority ethnic groups.

It is also essential that South Asian people with dementia are not seen as a peripheral group, with special, separate needs in terms of policy and practice. Along with other people with dementia for example, they need to be included in care standards guidance, currently the object of extended discussion in Scotland. Standard documents on community care are relevant for this group. They include, for example, the Commission for Racial Equality's guidelines for good practice in community care (CRE 1997), which offer an audit-based starting point for the identification of good practice in dementia-specific community care services for South Asian people. Inclusion of people with dementia in policy and practice needs to be part of the mainstreaming agenda.

Recent developments in research on dementia have prompted a focus on the person with dementia as a social actor (Downs 1997), and eliciting the perspective of the person with dementia is a growing concern across a variety of service settings (Downs 1997; Keady 1996). In research, such a focus requires the development of methodologies that can ascertain the perspectives and experiences of people formerly thought incapable of expressing them. New approaches promise to develop insights into the experiences of people with dementia that may inform the development of service provision (Duckett and Fryer 1997; Kitwood 1997), as well as wider efforts to promote social inclusion and address issues of exclusion based on ageism and disability. In doing so, they can privilege the perspective of the person with dementia, and approach issues of quality of life from this perspective, rather than through professionally defined measures (cf. Bland 1997). The South Asian person with dementia requires even greater sensitivity on the part of both researchers and service providers, but must nevertheless be included in research in the same way as others.

Conclusion

Thus, researchers attempting to ascertain the views of South Asian people with dementia face many problems in identifying appropriate research methods. As we have discussed, these include a dearth of previous research, few background statistics, issues of diagnosis, problems of identifying and contacting respondents, issues attached to the social identity of researchers and respondents, and problems with gaining informed consent.

But there are also many resources that researchers can use to advance work in this area. Other areas of research with South Asian people and with people with dementia offer many useful insights, which can inform the development of work with South Asian people with dementia. The key sources of relevant research are work on older people, on mental health issues and on disability. Research with South Asian people with dementia does not have to start from scratch.

Another key resource in developing this work lies in the practical experience of those who already work with South Asian people with dementia. Many of these will be South Asian community workers, mental health workers, social workers and so on, employed in specialist community projects, which do not necessarily focus on people with dementia, but to which they, or their families and carers, may come. It is important to identify ways of collecting data on this practical experience, identifying examples of best practice and disseminating these to others working in the field.

At times, the difficulties involved in working with South Asian people with dementia may appear insurmountable, because of all the problems we have discussed here. But we would suggest that the most useful ways forward will entail collaboration between researchers and people working closely with South Asian people with dementia in the communities. The key role of the researchers must be in deepening understanding of the condition of dementia, people's needs for services and support, which may or may not be distinctive, and the dissemination of good practice. To achieve these ends, the most useful research methodologies are likely to involve forms of collaborative and action research.

Notes

1. Mini-mental state examination – a psychometric screening tool that provides an overall quantitive estimate of cognitive impairment (Folstein, Folstein and McHugh 1975).

2. Other studies have used more expensive methods, such as identifying South Asian names from patient registers (Lindesay *et al.* 1997b; Rait *et al.* 2000). To identify people who have a diagnosis of dementia, large numbers have to be screened from such lists. Boneham *et al.*'s (1997) identification of one Indian person who possibly had dementia or depression from an initial list of 609 people aged 65 and over from minority ethnic groups in Liverpool indicates how complex such an approach can prove.

References

10/66 Dementia Research Group (2000a) 'Dementia in developing countries: A consensus statement from the 10/66 Dementia Research Group.' *International Journal of Geriatric Psychiatry 15*,14–20.

10/66 Dementia Research Group (2000b) 'Methodological issues for population-based research into dementia in developing countries: A position paper from the 10/66 Dementia Research Group.' *International Journal of Geriatric Psychiatry 15*, 21–30.

Ahmad, W. I. U. (1996) 'Family obligations and social change among Asian communities.' In W. I. U. Ahmad and K. Atkin (eds) *'Race' and Community Care*, pp.51-72. Buckingham: Open University Press.

Ahmod, W. I. U. and Atkin, K. (1996) (eds) *'Race' and Community Care*. Introduction. Buckingham: Open University Press.

Ahmad, W. I. U. and Walker, R. (1997) 'Asian older people: Housing, health and access to services.' *Ageing and Society 17*,141–165.

Allan, K. (2001) *Communication and Consultation: Exploring Ways for Staff to Involve People with Dementia in Developing Services.* Bristol: Policy Press.

Anderson, I. and Brownlie, J. (1997) 'A neglected problem: Minority ethnic elders with dementia.' In A. M. Bowes and D. F. Sim (eds) *Perspectives on Welfare: the Experience of Minority Ethnic Groups in Scotland.* Aldershot: Ashgate.

Atkin, K. and Rollings, J. (1993) *Community Care in a Multi-Racial Britain: A Critical Review of the Literature.* London: HMSO.

Azmi, S., Hatton, C., Emerson, E. and Caine, A. (1996) *Asian Staff in Services for People with Learning Disabilities.* Manchester: Hester Adrian Research Centre.

Azmi, S., Hatton, C., Emerson, E. and Caine, A. (1997) 'Listening to adolescents and adults with intellectual disabilities from South Asian communities.' *Journal of Applied Research in Intellectual Disabilities 10*, 3, 250–263.

Baker, F. M. (1996) 'Issues in assessing dementia in African American elders.' In G. Yeo and D. Gallagher-Thompson (eds) *Ethnicity and the Dementias*, pp.59–76 Washington DC: Taylor and Francis.

Bignall, T. and Butt, J. (2000) *Between Ambition and Achievement: Young Black Disabled People's Views and Experiences of Independence and Independent Living.* Bristol: Policy Press.

Blakemore, K. (2000) 'Health and social care needs in minority ethnic communities: An over-problematized issue?' *Health and Social Care in the Community 8*,1, 22–30.

Blakemore, K. and Boneham, M. (1994) *Age, Race and Ethnicity: A Comparative Approach.* Buckingham: Open University Press.

Bland, R. (1997) 'User-centred performance indicators for inspection of community care in Scotland: Developing a framework.' In A. Evers, R. Haverinen, K. Leischsenring and G. Wistow (eds) *Developing Quality in Personal Social Services.* Public Policy and Welfare Series, vol. 22. Aldershot: Ashgate.

Boneham, M. A., Williams, K. E., Copeland, J. R. M., McKibbin, P., Wilson, K., Scott, A. and Saunders, P. A. (1997) 'Elderly people from ethnic minorities in Liverpool: Mental illness, unmet need and barriers to service use.' *Health and Social Care in the Community 5*, 3, 173–180.

Bowes, A. M. and Dar, N. S. (1996) *Pathways to Welfare for Pakistani Elderly People in Glasgow.* Edinburgh: Central Research Unit, Scottish Office.

Bowes, A. M. and Dar, N. S. (2000) *Family Support and Community Care: A Study of South Asian Older People.* Edinburgh: Central Research Unit, Scottish Executive.

Bowes, A. M. and MacDonald, C. (2000) *Support for Majority and Minority Ethnic Groups at Home: Older People's Perspectives.* (Social Work Research Findings No. 36). Edinburgh: Scottish Executive Central Research Unit.

Bowes, A. M., Sim, D. F. and Srivastava, A. (2001) *Meeting the Support Needs of Black and Minority Ethnic Communities in Glasgow.* Edinburgh: Scottish Homes.

Brownfoot, J. (1998) *The Needs of People with Dementia and their Carers within Three Ethnic Minority Groups in Haringey.* London: Haringey Housing and Social Services and the London Regional Office of the Alzheimer's Disease Society.

Brownlie, J. (1991) *A Hidden Problem? Dementia Among Minority Ethnic Groups.* Stirling: Dementia Services Development Centre, University of Stirling.

Butt, J. and Mirza, K. (1996) *Social Care and Black Communities.* London: Race Equality Unit

Carlin, H. (1999) *'If I Had No Choice': The Housing Needs of Ethnic Elders.* Edinburgh: Age Concern Scotland.

Commission for Racial Equality (1997) *Race, Culture and Community Care: An Agenda for Action.* London: Commission for Racial Equality.

Department of Health Social Services Inspectorate (1998) *They Look After Their Own, Don't They? Inspection of Community Care Services for Black and Ethnic Minority Older People.* London: Department of Health.

Donaghy, E. (1997) 'Understanding depression in young South Asian women in Scotland.' In A.M. Bowes and D.F. Sim (eds) *Perspectives on Welfare: the Experience of Minority Ethnic Groups in Scotland.* Aldershot: Ashgate.

Downs, M. (1996) 'The role of general practice and the primary care team in dementia diagnosis and management.' *International Journal of Geriatric Psychiatry 11,* 11, 937–942.

Downs, M. (1997) 'The emergence of the person in dementia research.' *Ageing and Society 17,* 597–607.

Downs, M. and Marshall, M. (1997) *Dementia* (SNAP report). Glasgow: Scottish Forum for Public Health Medicine.

Duckett, P. and Fryer, D. (1997) 'Developing empowering research practices with people who have learning disabilities.' *Journal of Community and Applied Social Psychology 8,* 1, 57–65.

Folstein, M. F., Folstein, S. E. and McHugh, P. R. (1975) 'Minimental state examination: A practical method for grading the cognitive status of patients for the clinician.' *International Journal of Geriatric Psychiatry 10,* x, 687–194.

Ganguli, M., Ratcli, G., Chandra, V., Sharma, S., Gilby, J., Pandav, R., Belle, S., Ryan, C., Baker, C., Seaberg, E. and Dekosky, S. (1995) 'A Hindi version of the MMSE: The development of a cognitive screening instrument for a largely illiterate population in India.' *International Journal of Geriatric Psychiatry 10,* 367–377.

Huismann, A., Raven, U. and Geiger, A. (eds) (1998) *Neurodegenerative Diseases Among Migrants in EU States: Prevalence and Care Situation.* Bonn: Wissenschaftliches Institut der Ärzte Deutschlands e.V.

Kabir, Z. N. and Herlitz, A. (2000) 'The Bangla adaptation of Mini-Mental State Examination (BAMSE): An instrument to assess cognitive function in illiterate and literate individuals.' *International Journal of Geriatric Psychiatry 15*, 441–450.

Keady, J. (1996) 'The experience of dementia: a review of the literature and implications for nursing practice.' *Journal of Clinical Nursing 5*, 275–288.

Kitwood, T. (1997) *Dementia Reconsidered: The Person Comes First.* Buckingham: Open University Press.

Kvale, S. (1996) *InterViews: An Introduction to Qualitative Research Interviewing* Londaon: Sage.

Larson, E. B. and Imai, Y. (1996) 'An overview of dementia and ethnicity with special emphasis on the epidemiology of dementia.' In G. Yeo and D. Gallagher-Thompson (eds) *Ethnicity and the Dementias*, pp.9–20. Washington DC: Taylor and Francis.

Lindesay, J., Jagger, C., Hibbett, M. J., Peet, S. M. and Moledina, F. (1997a) 'Knowledge uptake and availability of health and social services among Asian and non-Asian elders.' *Ethnicity and Health 2*, 1–2, 59–69.

Lindesay, J., Jagger, C., Mlynik-Szmid, A., Sinorwala, A., Peet, S. and Moledina, F. (1997b) 'The Mini-Mental State Examination (MMSE) in an elderly immigrant Gujarati population in the United Kingdom.' *International Journal of Geriatric Psychiatry 12*, 1155–1167.

Marshall, M. (1999) 'What do service planners and policy makers need from research?' *International Journal of Geriatric Psychiatry 14*, 86–96.

Modood, T. and Berthoud, R., with Lakey, J., Nazroo, J., Smith, P., Virdee, S. and Beishon, S. (1997) *Ethnic Minorities in Britain: Diversity and Disadvantage.* London: Policy Studies Institute.

Mungas, D. (1996) 'The process of development of valid and reliable neuropsychological assessment measures for English- and Spanish-speaking elderly persons.' In G. Yeo and D. Gallagher-Thompson (eds) *Ethnicity and the Dementias*, pp.33–46. Washington DC: Taylor and Francis.

Nazroo, J. Y. (1997) *The Health of Britain's Ethnic Minorities.* London: Policy Studies Institute.

Nazroo, J. Y. (1999) *Ethnicity and Mental Health: Findings from a National Community Survey.* London: Policy Studies Institute.

Netto, G. (1996) *No-one Asked Us Before: Assessing the Needs of Minority Ethnic Carers of Older People in Edinburgh and the Lothians.* Edinburgh: SEMRU, Edinburgh College of Art/Heriot Watt University.

Netto, G. (1997) '"No-one has asked us before": The welfare needs of minority ethnic carers of older people in Lothian.' In A.M. Bowes and D.F. Sim (eds) *Perspectives on Welfare: the Experience of Minority Ethnic Groups in Scotland.* 135–150. Aldershot: Ashgate.

Norman, A. (1985) *Triple Jeopardy: Growing Old in a Second Homeland.* London: Centre for Policy on Ageing.

Parker, G. and Lawton, D. (1994) *Different Types of Care, Different Types of Carer: Evidence from the General Household Survey.* London: HMSO.

Patel, N., Mirza, N. R., Lindblad, P., Amstrup, K. and Samaoli, O. (1998) *Dementia and Minority Ethnic Older People: Managing Care in the UK, Denmark and France.* London: Russell House.

Pilgrim, D. and Rogers, A. (1999) *A Sociology of Mental Health and Illness.* Buckingham: Open University Press.

Rait, G., Burns, A., Baldwin, R., Morley, M., Chew-Graham, C. and St Leger, S. (2000) 'Validating screening instruments for cognitive impairment in older South Asians in the United Kingdom.' *International Journal of Geriatric Psychiatry 15,* 54–62.

Reid-Howie Associates (2001) *Review of Funding for Black and Minority Ethnic Groups in the Voluntary Sector.* Edinburgh: Scottish Executive.

Rhodes, P. (1994) 'Race-of-interviewer effects: A brief comment.' *Sociology 28,* 2, 547–558.

Sashidharan, S. P. and Francis, E. (1993) 'Epidemiology, ethnicity and schizophrenia.' In W. I. U. Ahmad (ed) *'Race' and Health In Contemporary Britain.* Buckingham: Open University Press.

Shah, A. (1999) 'Difficulties experienced by a Gujarati geriatric psychiatrist in interviewing Gujarati elders in Gujarati.' *International Journal of Geriatric Psychiatry 14,* 1072–1074.

Simpson, S. (1996) 'Non-response to the 1991 Census: The effect on ethnic group enumeration.' In D. Coleman and J. Salt *Ethnicity in the 1991 Census: Demographic Characteristics of the Ethnic Minority Populations.* London: HMSO.

Srivastava, A. and Bowes, A. M. (1996) *Mental Health among Elderly South Asians: A Review in the Light of Mental Health Services in Scotland.* Edinburgh: Scottish Office Home and Health Department, Chief Scientist Office.

Taussig, I. M. and Pontón, M. (1996) 'Issues in neuropsychological assessment for Hispanic older adults: Cultural and linguistic factors.' In G. Yeo and D. Gallagher-Thompson (eds) *Ethnicity and the Dementias.,* pp.47–58. Washington DC: Taylor and Francis.

Teng, E. L. (1996) 'Cross-cultural testing and the cognitive abilities screening instrument.' In G. Yeo and D. Gallagher-Thompson (eds) *Ethnicity and the Dementias,* pp.77–83. Washington DC: Taylor and Francis.

Tsolaki, M., Iakovidou, V., Navrozidou, H., Aminta, M., Panzati, T. and Kazis, A. (2000) 'Hindi mental state examination (HMSE) as a screening tool for illiterate demented patients.' *International Journal of Geriatric Psychiatry 15,* 662–665.

Twigg, J. (1992) *Carers: Research and Practice.* London: HMSO.

Yeo, G., Gallagher-Thompson, D. and Lieberman, M. (1996) 'Variations in dementia characteristics by ethnic category.' In G. Yeo and D. Gallagher-Thompson (eds) *Ethnicity and the Dementias,* pp.21–28. Washington DC: Taylor and Francis.

List of Contributors

Kate Allan's background is in clinical psychology where she worked in the field of mental health with adults and older adults. She is now Research Fellow at the Dementia Services Development Centre, University of Stirling, where she has been undertaking research in the area of communication and service user consultation.

Claire Bamford is a Senior Research Associate at the Centre for Health Services Research, University of Newcastle, where she is researching the use of primary care services by people with dementia. She previously worked on the Outcomes Programme at the Social Policy Research Unit, University of York, where she consulted a range of stakeholders, including older people with dementia, about the desired outcomes of social care. Her research interests include the experience of living with dementia, consulting hard-to-reach users and using an outcomes-focus to evaluate services.

Helen Bartlett is Foundation Director and Professor at the Centre for Human Ageing, University of Queensland. She worked at Oxford Brookes University from 1995 to 2001 in the School of Health Care as Professor of Health Studies, Deputy Head (Research) and Director of the Oxford Centre for Health Care Research and Development. During 1998/9 she was one of the founding co-directors of the Oxford Dementia Centre and continues as a research associate of the Centre. Her research has focused on quality measurement and policy issues in long-term care, in particular nursing and residential homes. These interests have been pursued in Asia, including Hong Kong, Taiwan and Japan. She is also an experienced health services researcher and has been involved in evaluating a range of primary health care services, including services for older people.

Alison Bowes is Professor of Sociology in the Department of Applied Social Science at the University of Stirling. She specialises in researching minority ethnic access to social work, housing and health services, with particular references to older people and women.

Errollyn Bruce is a part-time worker with Bradford Dementia Group. She is currently working on well-being in long term care. Previous work in the dementia field includes developing a supportive education approach for carers, and evaluating 'Remembering Yesterday, Caring Today', a reminiscence project working with carers and people with dementia together.

Charlotte Clarke has been active in dementia care research for more than a decade, with work focusing on the effect of health care intervention on families, the evaluation of innovative services and the exploration of clinical decision-making in continence care for older people with mental health needs. At present, Charlotte leads a research programme about practice development and works very closely with a number of health care providers. She has published a number of items about dementia care, including an edited book with Trevor Adams *(Dementia Care: Developing Partnerships in Practice*, 1999).

Ailsa Cook is a postgraduate research student in the Department of Applied Social Science at the University of Stirling. Her thesis is exploring the ways in which people with dementia manage their communicative experiences in two service settings. Prior to starting her PhD Ailsa was a research assistant at the Centre for Social Research on Dementia at the University of Stirling.

Lynne Corner is an Alzheimer's Society Research Fellow and is based at the Centre for Health Services Research and Institute for Ageing and Health, University of Newcastle upon Tyne. Dr Corner has a background in health services research for older people and a particular interest in the health and social care of older people with dementia and their carers.

Murna Downs was appointed as Professor in Dementia Studies and Head of Bradford Dementia Group at the University of Bradford in 2000. She has been working in the field of dementia for over ten years. She received her PhD in psychology at the University of Vermont and was awarded a National Institute of Mental Health postdoctoral fellowship in mental health and ageing at the Pennsylvania State University. She worked in the Department of Applied Social Science at the University of Stirling for six years, initially as Research Manager within the Dementia Services Development Centre and later as Director of the Centre for Social Research on Dementia. Her research interests centre on quality of life and quality of care for people with dementia and their families. She has published on a range of topics, including the role of primary care, diagnosis disclosure, nursing home care, dementia in a social and cultural context, and the place of the person in dementia research. She is a member of the Medical and Scientific Advisory Panel of the Alzheimer's Society (UK) and of the British Society of Gerontology Executive. Current collaborative research projects include a study of quality of life in nursing homes.

Gill Hubbard is currently Research Fellow at University of Stirling for an ESRC-funded project on exploring quality of life of frail older people. She is an experienced researcher who has worked with vulnerable groups of people in a variety of settings. Her interests include developing guidelines for research teams working with vulnerable groups of people and the management of sensitive and emotional issues.

John Keady is Senior Lecturer in the School of Nursing and Midwifery at the University of Wales, Bangor. John's main research interests are in the subjective experience of dementia, carers and coping and in training issues around dementia care.

Wendy Martin is Research Fellow at the Oxford Dementia Centre for a two-year funded project entitled 'Empowering older people with dementia: balancing rights, risk and choice in different care settings'. She qualified as a Registered General Nurse in 1986 at St Mary's School of Nursing, London, and her clinical background includes working in both acute and cancer care specialities. In 1997 she completed a BSc in Sociology and Anthropology at Oxford Brookes University, followed by an MA in Sociological Research in Health Care at Warwick University. She has previously held positions as a researcher on projects relating to ageing, cancer care and family studies.

Anne Mason is Research Fellow in the Centre for Social Research on Dementia at the University of Stirling. Her current research is focused around the legal needs and experiences of people with dementia in Scotland. As a qualified nurse educator, Anne has a diversity of experience within the statutory and voluntary sectors. Her main interests and experiences are concerned with the psycho-social needs of people with mental health problems, particularly older people.

Rebekah Pratt worked for the Centre for Social Research on Dementia, University of Stirling, Scotland, on a project looking at the experience of people with dementia in relation to diagnosis disclosure. Rebekah is a New Zealand-trained community psychologist with a background in family violence, health, drugs and alcohol and evaluation research.

Susan Tester is a principal investigator for an ESRC-funded project on exploring quality of life of frail older people. She is currently a Senior Lecturer in social policy at the University of Stirling, where she specialises in community care, ageing, and comparative social policy, with a particular interest in Europe. Her recent research includes coordinating a transnational study of institutional care in collaboration with Alzheimer Scotland - Action on Dementia and Alzheimer organisations in the Netherlands, Italy and Spain. Her publications include *Community Care for Older People: a comparative perspective*, *Common Knowledge: a coordinated approach to information giving*, and *Caring by Day: a study of day care services for older people*.

Heather Wilkinson is a Research Fellow in the Centre for Social Research on Dementia and the Royal Society of Edinburgh Lloyds TSB Personal Research Fellow from January 2001–2004. Heather's current research interests include legal and ethical issues for people with dementia; the experience of dementia for people from ethnic minority groups; and people with learning difficulties and dementia. Heather works within a social model framework that places the person with dementia at the centre.

Subject index

absent-mindedness 32
accessing participants and gaining consent
  58–9
action checklists 28
Action on Dementia *see under* Alzheimer
  Scotland
Adults with Incapacity (Scotland) Act 2000 9,
  66–7, 183, 184, 188
advance consent directives 51–2, 65–6, 68
advisory networks and user panels 83–97
  benefits of user panel to research 94–5
  consumer involvement 83–4
  establishing user panel 86–7
  form of user panel 87–9
  how have panel members found the
    process? 92–4
  involving people with dementia in user
    panel 84
  log of activities over 12 weeks 89
  phases of research project 85
  purpose of user panel 84–6
  what does panel do? 90
ageism 9, 236
agitation 31
alcohol abuse 184
  misdiagnosis of 103
Alzheimer's disease (AD) 32, 58, 93, 112,
  169, 170, 178, 184, 200
  should people with Alzheimer's take part
    in research? 101–7
Alzheimer Scotland 102, 106, 110, 111, 112,
  187
  Action on Dementia (ASAD) 110, 111,
    112–13, 187, 205
Alzheimer's Society 84, 86
Alzheimer's Society of India 230
ambiguities and problems with consent 143–4
American Geriatrics Society 65, 68
anti-depressants 101
anti-Alzheimer medication 29, 178
anxiety 33, 36, 37, 41, 51, 93
Arthur's Seat, Edinburgh 106
assent, seeking 52–3
assessment 27, 64–5
  of competency 53–4
attitudes encountered by James 114
autonomy 13

baby talkers (attitude encountered by James)
  114
Bangladesh(is) 228, 230, 233
BASOLL *see* Behavioural Scale of Later Life
BBC 106
behavioural consent 66
Behavioural Scale of Later Life (BASOLL) 56
beneficence 49

bi-polar disorders 184
Bradford Dementia Group 30
Brenda (worker at Turning Point) 111
British Psychological Society 68
British Society of Gerontology 68
British Sociological Association 68
  Code of Ethical Practice 235

cannots (attitude encountered by James) 114
caregiving 34
care home managers 27, 57
care home residents 54
carers 26, 34, 55, 86–8, 92, 143, 199
  role of 168–9
case records, analysis of 55
challenging behaviour 56, 119
children 37, 39–40
clinical research 47
coercion 57
cognitive abilities 16–17
cognitive behaviour therapy 31
cognitive difficulties 195–6
cognitive impairment 51
cognitive screening 30, 31
collaboration vs. control 127–8
collaborative approach to data collection 35,
  41
Comic Relief 106
Commission for Racial Equality (CRE) 236
common sense approach to research 49
Communication and Consultation (Allan) 117
communication difficulties 71
community
  care 55
  psychiatric nurses (CPNs) 32, 143, 186–7,
    190, 202–3, 204
  psychology methodology 166
competency
  assessment of 53–4
  intermittent 65, 78
  lack of 51
comprehension difficulties 71
computers 105, 198
concerned (attitude encountered by James)
  114
confidence 131
confidentiality 135, 145, 203
  agreement 53
  and openness 198–200
confusion 31, 104
consent 58, 87, 119, 211–14, 234–5
  ambiguities and problems with 143–4
  behavioural 66
  continuous 67
  form 70–1
  informed 38, 48, 50–3, 63–4, 68, 70, 71,
    73–5, 77, 78, 87
  monitoring 79
  negotiated 66
  process and perspectives of older people in
    institutional care 63–80
    assessment 64–5

case examples 72–7
    gathering consent during research
        69–77
    strategies 65–8
    proxy 66, 68, 69, 75, 76, 79
    seeking 142–3
consumer(s)
    individuals as 13
    involvement 83–4
context, significance of 153–5
continuous consent 67
control vs. collaboration 127–8
counselling 30, 192, 196
creating mental picture 201–2
creativity 40
credibility of data 37
culture and language, issues of 233–4

data
    collection 25–41, 69
        early steps 31–4
        quality 34–40
day care 118
    managers 58
daydreams 32
DCM see Dementia Care Mapping
deafness 87
decision-making
    capacity 58
        fluctuations in 65
    pathways 55
    surrogate 65
deliberative approach 140
Dementia Care Mapping (DCM) 30, 39, 209
demographic data 191, 224
depression 31, 184, 229, 230
detachment of interviewer 38
developing understanding 12–15
diagnosis of dementia 102–3, 104, 107, 110,
    113, 232
    early 29
diary 91
disability 236
    esearch 12
discriminatory practices 189
distress 54, 66, 78
    dealing with 171–2
'does he take sugar' (attitude encountered by
    James) 114
double consents 58
drugs 84
duration of interviews 37, 51

early dementia (Early Onset Dementia) 31-40,
    106
early diagnosis of dementia 29
early memory loss 36
easy-access memory board 40
Economic and Social Research Council
    Qualidata 65
Edinburgh City Hospital 101

effective therapeutic intervention 26
emancipatory research 12
emotional content 194
empathy 33, 192, 198
empowerment 13, 47, 58
    lessons from study of 55–9
        accessing participants and gaining
            consent 58–9
        issues in negotiating gatekeepers 55–8
        overview 55
epidemiological data 224
ethical issues 19, 47–60, 218–20
ethical principles 48–50
ethics committees 58, 69, 71, 79, 202
ethnic minorities 225, 226
evidence-based specialist care 28
exclusion 15

facial muscles, stiffening of 105
familiarity 151–3
family members 52, 53, 55–8
feedback 106, 130–1
    exercise 133–4
feminist research 12, 166
focus groups 17
    background 140–2
    focus and interaction in 146–50
        achieving focus 147–8
        generating interaction between 148–50
    with older people with dementia
        distinctive features of 150–61
            background information about
                participants 155
            domination by one or two participants
                155–6
            familiarity 151–3
            idealised accounts 157–9
            interpreting data 160–1
            parallel conversations 156–7
            significance of context 153–5
            storytelling 159–60
        issues in using 151
    potential advantages of 141
    practical issues in convening and running
        141–6
        ambiguities and problems with consent
            143–4
        confidentiality 145
        exercising choice over participation
            144–5
        identifying potential participants 141–2
        inviting participation and seeking
            consent 142–3
        organising and running 145–6
    successes and challenges in using with
        older people with dementia 139–
        62
    topic guide and case study 146
forgetfulness 31, 32, 174, 196
formal advance consent directives 66
Fourth National Survey of Ethnic Minorities in
    Britain 233

funding 33, 87

gatekeepers 55–8, 167, 211–12, 221, 232
general practitioners (GPs) 29, 32, 103, 104,
    107, 186, 229
Glasgow 232
gloom merchants (attitude encountered by
    James) 114
groups
    discussion 88, 119, 145, 153
    focus see focus groups
    informal 154–5
    mixed 88
    vulnerable 173
Guidelines for Good Practice in Telephone Work
    192
Gujarati 226

health board ethics committees 69
health care professionals 55, 56, 58, 78, 85
Health of a Nation (white paper, DoH, 1992)
    28
health service provision 26
Hearing the Voice of People with Dementia
    (Goldsmith) 117
Henry, Lenny 106
Hispanic Americans 225
home, research studies taking place in own 34
home care 140, 147
    managers 57, 58, 70, 71, 75
honesty 198
hospital admissions 39
Hughes Hall Project for Later Life 33–4

idealised accounts 157–9
inattention 31
inclusion of people with dementia in research
    9–20
incompetence 53
incredibles (attitude encountered by James)
    114
India(ns) 224, 225, 230, 233
infantilisation 70
informal groups 154–5
informed consent 38, 48, 50–3, 63–4, 68, 70,
    71, 73–5, 77, 78, 87,
    173–5
infringing on privacy 53
insecurity 51
institutional care, perspectives during consent
    process of older people
in 63–80
interactions
    in focus groups 146–50, 161
        generating between participants 148–50
    with participants, reviewing 215–17
    recording 214–15
interactional abilities 16
intermediate care 28
intermittent competency 65, 78

internal preoccupation with thoughts and
    daydreams 32
interpersonal skills 192
interpretative abilities 16
interpreting data 160–1
intervention, effective therapeutic 26
interviews 33–9, 57, 85, 90, 102, 110
    and feelings of people with dementia
        165–81
        allowing time 176–7
        creating safe contexts 166–72
            dealing with distress 171–2
            gatekeepers 167
            questioner becomes questioned 169–71
            role of carers 168–9
        developing reflective practice 177–9
            supervision 178–9
        informed consent 173–5
        and interviewee safety 179–80
        key points 167, 169, 171, 173, 175–7,
            179, 181
        matters of method 175–6
    by telephone 183–205
    timing of 34

key principles regarding people with dementia
    (King's Fund Centre
report) 26–7
knowledgeable (attitude encountered by
    James) 114

language
    and culture, issues of 233–4
    problems 32
    skills 36
Law Commission report (1993) 48, 51
learning difficulties/disabilities 36, 52, 229
life review approaches 31
listening and responding skills 192–200
    cognitive difficulties 195–6
    emotional content 194
    openness and confidentiality 198–200
    personal attributes 194–5
    personal values 200
    terminology 197
    willingness to participate 197–8
literature search and review 85
lived experience, dementia as 26–31
Local Research Ethics Committee (LREC) 49,
    55, 56, 57
location of data collection 37, 41
longitudinal studies 52
long-term nursing care settings 118
LREC see Local Research Ethics Committee

'malignant social psychology' 30
management 56
marginalisation 17
medicalisation of dementia 50
Medical Research Council 49, 52
memory 39, 56

change guidelines 30
clinics 30, 37
early loss of 36
failure 32
problems 52, 59, 71, 156, 232
therapy 30
mental illness 140, 228
mental picture, creating 201–2
middle management 56
Mini Mental State Examination (MMSE) 56, 175, 226
minority ethnic groups 225, 226
misdiagnosis of alcohol abuse 103
MMSE *see* Mini Mental State Examination
monitoring consent 79
monosyllabics (attitude encountered by James) 114
motor problems 32
multi-agency work 28
multidisciplinary team 40, 104
muscles, stiffening of facial 105
Muslims 230

name recall 174
narrative research 36
National Institute of Clinical Excellence 29
National Service Framework for Older People (NSF) 28–9
National Vocational Qualifications (NVQs) 192
negotiated consent 66
negotiating gatekeepers, issues in 55–8
negotiation 13, 58, 232
New Zealand 110
NHS and Community Care Act (DoH 1990) 27, 28, 183
non-maleficence 49
non-therapeutic research 49
non-verbal behaviours 71, 72
non-verbal communication 39, 119
non-verbal signals 66
NSF *see National Service Framework for Older People*
NUD*IST 72
nurses 31, 32, 119
nursing homes 69

observation 17, 39, 71, 75
observational data collection 39
obsessive behaviour 174
openness and confidentiality 198–200
organisational change 120
orientation 56

painkillers 101
Pakistan(is) 226, 228, 230, 233
parallel conversations 156–7
participant observation 55
participation 88
    exercising choice over 144–5

inviting 142–3
    and social relations 17
    willingness to participate 197–8
participatory research 95
Patient's Charter 28
personal attributes 194–5
personal values 200
person-centred approach 13, 14, 27, 30, 94
photographic chart 40
pilot studies 57
population and incidence of South Asians with dementia 224–7
poverty 229
power
    issues 196
    shifting 10–12
preventative action 26
primary care team 29
    nurses 31
privacy 199
    infringing on 53
    of people with dementia 58
process consent 38
professional care staff 55, 56, 58, 78, 85
promotion of active, healthy life 28
protective caregiving 36
proxy consent 54, 66, 68, 69, 75, 76, 78, 79
psychiatric nurses 119
psychiatrists 103
psycho-biography 32
psychogeriatricians 32
psycho-social intervention 30
psychotherapy 31, 184

QRD *see* Quality Research in Dementia
Quakers 106
qualitative interviews 90
qualitative research 51, 86, 90, 95
quality of life 63, 85, 86, 94
Quality Research in Dementia (QRD) 84
    Advisory Network 84
questioner becomes questioned 169–71
questionnaires 17, 133–4

racism 229
rapport 34, 177
reality orientation 31
Rebekah (researcher) 110–11, 113
recording
    interactions 214–15
    thoughts 105
reflective practice 177–9
relationships with staff, developing 121–3
relatives 33, 34, 57, 78
reliability of data 39, 41
researchers 72–7, 94–5, 105, 109
    what staff need from 128–31
residential care home 55, 69, 118
    manager 57, 70, 71, 75
resolution therapy 31
respect for individual 28, 198

responding
    quickly 130
    skills 193–200
rights
    of individual 13
    of people with dementia 58
    of vulnerable groups in research 48
risk-taking 33, 58
ritual 153
Royal Scottish Academy of Music and Drama
    220

safety 55
    creating safe contexts 166–72
    of interviewees 179–80
sample sizes, small 34
saying goodbye 202–3
Scandinavia 210
Scotland 69, 102, 185, 226, 228
screening test 54
seeking assent 52–3
self awareness 32
self care 16, 56
self esteem 36, 131
semi-structured interviews 17, 32
senior management 56
sensitivity 198
service providers 56
sheltered housing 55
shifting power 10–12
shift system 129
silences 200–1
skills 189
snowballing 148
social abilities 16
social inclusion 9, 15, 236
social isolation 36, 230
social model of disability 11
social psychology 30
social relations and participation 17
social research 25, 38, 47, 139
social work departments 69, 71
social workers 27, 32, 237
socio-political factors 50
South Asian people with dementia, research
        issues of 223–37
    current knowledge
        population and incidence 224–7
        relevant research 227–30
    research issues 231–5
        consent 234–5
        identifying respondents 231–3
        issues of language and culture 233–4
        ways forward for future research 235–6
stigma 9, 10
Stirling see University of Stirling
stories 31
storytelling 128, 159–60
    interpreting 160–1
stress 26, 93
structured interviews 17
supervision 178–9

support groups 30
surrogate decision-making 65

tape-recording
    of interviews 37–9
    of panel discussions 91
    of thoughts 105
telephone interviews with people with
        dementia 183–205
    background to study 185
    core skills required for 192–200
        listening and responding skills 193–200
    creating mental picture 201–2
    impact of interview and saying goodbye
        202–3
    main study 188–9
    pilot study 186
    silences 200–1
    structure of interview 191
    welcoming participant to interview
        189–91
terminology 197
therapeutic research 49
time, problems with 36
timing of interview 34
tiredness 37, 38, 41
TLC (tender loving care) 112
tokenism 86
transcription and analysis 217–18
transport problems 88
trust 33, 48, 196, 198
Turning Point Scotland 110, 111

unbelievers (attitude encountered by James)
    114
United Kingdom 14, 27, 28, 47, 102, 183,
    223–7, 230, 233
United States 16, 52, 58, 225
University of Stirling 102, 106, 205, 220,
    229
unresponsiveness 36
Urdu 226
user involvement 85
user panels
    and advisory networks 83–97
    benefits of, to research 94–5
    establishing 86–7
    form of 87–9
    how have panel members found the
        process? 92–4
    involving people with dementia in 84
    purpose of 84–6
    what do they do? 90

validation
    during interviews 38
    therapy 31, 141
verbal signals 66
veterans 16
video observation 209–21

    ethical issues 218–20
    recording interactions 214–15
    reviewing with participants 215–17
    starting out, negotiating access, gaining
        consent to do research 211–14
    transcription and analysis 217–18
voice of person with dementia 47
voluntary organisations 188
volunteers 53
vulnerable group 173

wardens 57
warmth 198
welcoming participant to interview 189–91
wellwishers (attitude encountered by James)
    114
whisperers (attitude encountered by James)
    114
willingness to participate 197–8
working with staff to include people with
    dementia in research 117–36
    control vs. collaboration 127–8
    developing relationships with staff 121–3
    finishing up 133–5
    feedback exercise 133–4
    written outcomes 134–5
    getting to know services 124–6
    helping staff to become aware of what they
        already know and do 123–4
    involving staff in design and carrying out
        of work 126–7
    project 117–21
    using our own experiences to enhance
        understanding of person with
dementia 132
    values inherent in the work 121
    what staff need from a researcher 128–31
      boosting self-esteem and confidence 131
      fitting in with their routines 129–30
      providing feedback 130–1
      responding quickly 130
workshop sessions 122
written outcomes 134–5

Author index

Acton, G.J. 32
Adams, T. 31, 47
Agarwal, M. 47, 48, 51, 53, 64
Ahmad, W.I.U. 224, 227, 228, 235
Allan, K. 80, 117–37, 234, 243
Alm, N. 184
Alzheimer, A. 17
Alzheimer's Disease Society 28
Alzheimer's Society 84, 97
American Geriatrics Society 64, 65, 68
Anderson, I. 33, 36, 223, 226
Aneshensel, C. 184
Appelbam, P. 64
Asplund, K. 31, 210
Athlin, E. 210
Atkin, K. 227, 235
Audit Commission 28, 29
Azmi, S. 229

Bach, 12
Baker, F.M. 227
Bamford, C. 18, 97, 139–64, 243
Banks-Wallace, J. 147, 150, 160
Barak, Y. 184
Barbour, R.S. 84, 139, 141, 151, 154
Barnes, C. 11, 13, 85
Barnett, E. 13, 17, 53, 118, 159, 160
Baron, S. 12
Bartlett, H. 18, 47–61, 142, 243
Baskin, S. 47, 65
Bastion, H. 83
Beech, L. 118, 161
Bell, P. 30
Bender, M. 11, 17, 147, 159, 160
Bennett, G. 63, 85
Bennett-Emslie, G. 85
Beresford, P. 9, 85
Berghmans, R. 47, 49, 51, 53, 64, 66
Bignall, T. 229
Bjorn, 187
Blakemore, K. 226, 227, 230
Bland, R. 236
Bleathman, C. 141
Bloor, M. 151, 152, 155
Bond, J. 47, 97
Boneham, M.A. 226, 230, 231, 237
Booth, T. 36, 39
Booth, W. 36, 39
Borell, L. 32
Bowers, B.J. 36
Bowes, A.M. 19, 223–41, 243
Bowie, P. 209
Brandt, J. 184
Bredin, K. 30, 192, 209
British Sociological Association 64, 68
Brody, E. 11

Brooker, D. 17, 30, 56
Browne, J. 63
Brownfoot, J. 225, 231
Brownlie, J. 223, 226
Bruce, E. 18, 19, 139–64, 243
Burchardt, T. 15
Butt, J. 227, 229
Byatt, S. 17
Bytheway, B. 12

Cantley, C. 39
Carlin, H. 227
Carr-Hill, R. 83
Challis, D. 27
Cheston, R. 11, 17, 30, 139, 147, 159, 160
Clare, L. 30
Clarke, C.L. 17, 25–46, 47, 50, 52, 244
Coen, R. 63
Cohen, D. 14
Cohen, M.B. 159
Cohen, ? 204
Collopy, B. 173
Commission for Racial Equality (CRE) 228, 236
Cook, A. 18, 209–22, 244
Corner, L. 18, 47, 83–98, 244
Cornwell, J. 144, 147, 157
Cotrell, V. 13, 15, 32, 34, 165, 183
Craig, M. 97
Croft, S. 85
Crossan, B. 47, 50, 51, 52, 67

Dabbs, C. 118
Dar, N.S. 226, 230, 231, 232
Das, R. 141
Datan, N. 9
David, P. 153
Davis, L.L. 184
Davis, R. 16, 17
Dawson, P. 16
Deatrick, J.A. 37
De Lepeleire, J. 29
Dementia Services Development Centre 58
Department of Health 13, 28, 118, 183, 228
Dickenson, D. 51
Dixon, P. 83
Doherty-Sneddon, G. 221
Donaghy, E. 228, 229, 230
Downs, M. 11, 13, 15, 16, 18, 29, 47, 63–82, 165, 232, 235, 236, 244
Duckett, P. 47, 166, 236
Duelli Klein, R. 12
Duff, G. 30
Dukoff, R. 65, 66

Ekman, S.L. 173
Ericson, P.K. 32

Farquhar, M. 69, 139, 141

Faux, S.A. 37
Feil, N. 31, 139
Field, P.A. 38
Filkin, G. 118
Fincham, F. 118
Fine, M. 219
Fisk, M. 54, 56
Fiske, M. 141
Folstein, M. 184, 237
Folstein, S.E. 237
Forbes, D. 63
Francis, E. 226
Frank, W. 63
Fortinsky, R.H. 29
French, S. 12
Froggatt, A. 32, 33
Fryer, D. 166, 236

Gallagher-Thompson, D. 31, 225
Ganguli, M. 227
Garrett, K.J. 159
Geiger, A. 225
Gibson, F. 139
Gilleard, C.J. 26, 27
Gilliard, J. 16, 32, 35, 47
Gillies, B. 16, 32
Gisser, N. 168
Goldsmith, M. 32, 47, 117, 118, 183
Goudie, F. 31
Green, J. 154, 155
Greenbaum, T.L. 152, 155, 156
Gregor, P. 184
Grisso, T. 64
Groggatt, A. 13
Gubrium, J. 48, 63
Gwyther, L.P. 93, 94

Haggstrom, T. 219
Hanley, B. 83
Hanson, E. 184
Harding, N. 11, 50
Harding, S. 9, 12
Harre, R. 10
Hart, L. 154, 155
Harvey, R. 30, 97
Health Advisory Service 26, 28
Heller, L. 157
Helmchen, H. 64
Herlitz, A. 227
Heyman, R. 37
Heyrman, J. 29
High, D. 47, 52, 54
HMSO 67
Hockey, J. 70
Holden, U.P. 31
Holloway, W. 165
Hubbard, G. 18, 63–82, 221, 245
Huismann, A. 225, 226
Hungler, B. 192
Husband, H.J. 173

Imai, Y. 225

Jack, R. 12
Jackson, D. 30
Jackson, R. 35
James, A. 70
Jansson, L. 210
Jarrett, R.L. 157
Jefferson, T. 165

Kabir, Z.N. 227
Kalisch, B. 192
Kayser-Jones, J. 47, 48, 51, 58, 142, 143
Keady, J. 15, 16, 17, 25–46, 47, 52, 184,
    236, 245
Kendall, P.L. 141
Kenyon, G. 48
Kilhgren, M. 210
King's Fund Centre 26, 27
Kitwood, T. 30, 50, 64, 68, 192, 209, 236
Kitzinger, C. 12
Kitzinger, J. 88, 139, 141, 151, 152, 154,
    157
Knapp, 14
Knight, B.G. 26
Knox, K. 35, 36, 39
Koch, T. 63
Koenig, B. 47, 48, 51, 58, 142, 143
Krueger, R.A. 139, 141, 150, 151, 155, 156,
    162
Kulman, G.J. 26
Kvale, S. 234

Lam, J. 118, 161
La Monica, E. 192
Larson, E.B. 225
La Rue, A. 31
Law Commission 48, 51
Lawton, D. 227, 228
Lee, R.M. 36
Le Grand, J. 15
Leighton, A. 29
Levy, R. 184
Lieberman, M. 225
Lindesay, J. 224, 225, 226, 237
Litherland, R. 97
Lord Chancellor's Department 48
Lutzky, S.M. 26
Lyman, K.A. 10, 13, 14, 16

McAfee, M.E. 30
McAuslane, L. 17, 118, 140, 153, 159, 161
McColgan, G. 47, 50, 51, 52, 67
Macdonald, A.M. 184
MacDonald, C. 235
McGee, H. 63
McGowin, D.F. 16
McHugh, P.R. 237
McKillop, J. 18, 19, 109–14, 210

McKinlay, A. 205
McKinnen, L. 97
McLaren, P. 184
Macofsky-Urban, F. 26
Manion, 204
Maquire, C.P. 168
Marquis, R. 35
Marshall, M. 235
Marson, D. 64, 65
Martin, G.W. 30
Martin, W. 18, 47–61, 142, 245
Mason, A. 15, 18, 19, 183–207, 245
Mason, J. 142, 143
Medical Research Council 48, 49, 52
Melin, E. 210
Merton, R.K. 141
Michell, L. 152
Miller, M. 48
Milne, A.J. 29
Mills, M. 10, 16
Mirza, K. 227, 229
Mishler, E.G. 188, 189, 193
Mitchell, P. 63
Modood, T. 233
Mok, M. 35
Moniz-Cook, E. 16, 30
Moore, E. 205
Morgan, D.L. 139, 141, 150, 157, 162
Morris, 15
Morse, J.M. 38
Morton, I. 141
Mountain, G. 209
Mungas, D. 225, 227
Murphy, E. 90

Nazroo, J.Y. 225, 226, 228
Netto, G. 228, 230
Norberg, A. 31, 210
Norman, A. 227, 228
Normann, H.K. 31
Nusberg, C. 9
Nygård, L. 32

Oakley, A. 155
O'Boyle, C. 63
O'Connor, D.W. 33
Oliver, M. 11
Orbach, A. 31

Page, S. 31
Palfrey, C. 11, 50
Parker, G. 227, 228
Parmenter, T.R. 35
Patel, N. 226
Payton, V.R. 10, 63, 66, 70
Peach, E. 30
Peiris, D. 184, 198
Phair, L. 118
Phillips, L.R. 210
Phinney, A. 32

Piachaud, D. 15
Pilgrim, D. 226
Pinner, G. 30
Plotkin, D.A. 31
Polit, D. 192
Pollitt, P.A. 33, 36
Pontón, M. 227
Post, S.G. 20
Pratt, R. 15, 16, 18, 165–82, 187, 209, 245
Priestley, M. 183
Proctor, G. 9, 11, 15, 118

Qualitative Solutions and Research 72
Qureshi, H. 140, 161

Rait, G. 226, 237
Raudonis, B.M. 38, 39
Ravdal, H. 146
Raven, U. 225
Raynes, N. 63
Reed, J. 10, 40, 63, 66, 70
Rees, J. 30
Reid-Howie Associates 232
Revicki, D.A. 184
Reynolds, W. 192
Rhodes, P. 233
Riddell, S. 12
Riger, S. 166, 177
Rioux, 12
Robinson, Dave 101–3, 105–7
Robinson, Elaine 18, 19, 101–7, 111, 210
Robinson, Gail 101
Robinson, P. 37, 173
Robinson, Paul 101
Rodeheaver, D. 9
Rogers, A. 226
Rollings, J. 227
Rosenfield, R. 189, 190, 192, 193, 198
Royal College of Physicians 26
Royal College of Psychiatrists 49
Ruh, P.A. 30

Sabat, S.R. 10, 11, 14, 20, 173
Sachs, G. 64, 65, 66
Sankar, A. 48
Sartain, S. 37, 39
Sashidharan, S.P. 226
Schoenberg, N.E. 146
Schulz, R. 13, 15, 32, 34, 165, 183
Schumm, J.S. 139
Shah, A. 51, 234
Shamdasani, P.N. 150, 162
Shewan, J. 184
Silber, E. 93
Sim, D.F. 230
Simpson, S. 224
Sinagub, J. 139
Slutske, W.S. 184
Smallwood, J. 17
Smith, M. 97, 141, 219

Snyder, L. 31
Social Services Inspectorate (SSI) 28, 228
Spalding, J. 63
Spencer, M. 184
Sperlinger, D. 17, 118, 140, 153, 159, 161
Splann Krothe, J. 63
Srivastava, A. 228, 229, 230
Stalker, K. 12, 16, 47, 52, 56, 58
Standing Advisory Group on Consumer
    Involvement 83
Stern, P.N. 32
Stewart, D.W. 150, 162
Stewart, J. 140
Stokes, G. 31
Sunderland, T. 65, 66, 93
Sutton, L.J. 31, 118
Swain, J. 12

Taussig, I.M. 227
Telephone Helplines Association 192
Teng, E.L. 227
Teri, L. 31
Ter Meulen, R. 47, 49, 51, 53, 64, 66
Tester, S. 18, 63–82, 221, 246
Tetley, J. 184
Thompson, N. 13
Thompson, S. 13
Thornton, P. 13, 95
Tozer, R. 13, 95
Trickey, H. 30
Tsolaki, M. 227
Twigg, J. 227

Van Haitsma, K. 209
Van Ort, S. 210
Vassilas, C. 167
Vaughn, S. 139, 148, 152, 156

Wahlund, L.O. 173
Walker, R. 224
Walmsley, J. 12, 18
Ward, T. 209
Wasson, J.H. 29
Watson, J. 31
Weaver-Moore, L. 48
Wells, D.L. 16
Welsh Office 28
Whitsed-Lipinska, D. 30
Wigley, V. 54, 56
Wilkinson, H. 9–23, 107, 111, 113, 114,
    166, 171, 173–7, 181, 183–
    07, 209, 221, 223–41, 246
Williams, B. 198
Williams, J. 30
Winner, M. 27
Wistow, G. 85
Wonson, S. 30
Woods, B. 31
Woods, R.T. 31
Wuest, J. 32

Yale, R. 30, 139
Yeo, G. 225
Younger, D. 30